HOW TO
LIVE LONGER

BOOKS BY VERNON COLEMAN

The Medicine Men (1975)
Paper Doctors (1976)
Everything You Want To Know About Ageing (1976)
Stress Control (1978)
The Home Pharmacy (1980)
Aspirin or Ambulance (1980)
Face Values (1981)
Guilt (1982)
The Good Medicine Guide (1982)
Stress And Your Stomach (1983)
Bodypower (1983)
An A to Z Of Women's Problems (1984)
Bodysense (1984)
Taking Care Of Your Skin (1984)
A Guide to Child Health (1984)
Life Without Tranquillisers (1985)
Diabetes (1985)
Arthritis (1985)
Eczema and Dermatitis (1985)
The Story Of Medicine (1985, 1998)
Natural Pain Control (1986)
Mindpower (1986)
Addicts and Addictions (1986)
Dr Vernon Coleman's Guide To Alternative Medicine (1988)
Stress Management Techniques (1988)
Overcoming Stress (1988)
Know Yourself (1988)
The Health Scandal (1988)
The 20 Minute Health Check (1989)
Sex For Everyone (1989)
Mind Over Body (1989)
Eat Green Lose Weight (1990)
Why Animal Experiments Must Stop (1991)
The Drugs Myth (1992)
How To Overcome Toxic Stress (1991)
Why Doctors Do More Harm Than Good (1993)
Stress and Relaxation (1993)
Complete Guide To Sex (1993)
How to Conquer Backache (1993)
Betrayal of Trust (1994)

How to Conquer Pain (1994)
Know Your Drugs (1994, 1997)
Food for Thought (1994)
The Traditional Home Doctor (1994)
I Hope Your Penis Shrivels Up (1994)
People Watching (1995)
Relief from IBS (1995)
The Parent's Handbook (1995)
Oral Sex: Bad Taste And Hard To Swallow? (1995)
Why Is Pubic Hair Curly? (1995)
Men in Dresses (1996)
Power over Cancer (1996)
Crossdressing (1996)
How To Get The Best Out Of Prescription Drugs (1996)
How To Get The Best Out of Alternative Medicine (1996)
How To Conquer Arthritis (1996)
High Blood Pressure (1996)
How To Stop Your Doctor Killing You (1996)
Fighting For Animals (1996)
Alice and Other Friends (1996)
Dr Coleman's Fast Action Health Secrets (1997)
Dr Vernon Coleman's Guide to Vitamins and Minerals (1997)
Spiritpower (1997)
Other People's Problems (1998)
How To Publish Your Own Book (1999)
How To Relax and Overcome Stress (1999)
Animal Rights – Human Wrongs (1999)
Superbody (1999)
The 101 Sexiest, Craziest, Most Outrageous
   Agony Column Questions (and Answers) of All Time (1999)
Strange but True (2000)
How To Make Money While Watching TV (2000)
Food for Thought [revised edition] (2000)
Daily Inspirations (2000)
Stomach Problems: Relief At Last (2001)
How To Overcome Guilt (2001)
Animal Rights – Human Wrongs Pocket Edition (2001)

reports

Prostate Trouble (2000)
Vitamins and Minerals (2000)
How To Campaign (2000)

Genetic Engineering (2000)
Osteoporosis (2000)
Vaccines (2000)
Alternative Medicine (2000)

novels

The Village Cricket Tour (1990)
The Bilbury Chronicles (1992)
Bilbury Grange (1993)
Mrs Caldicot's Cabbage War (1993)
Bilbury Revels (1994)
Deadline (1994)
The Man Who Inherited a Golf Course (1995)
Bilbury Country (1996)
Second Innings (1999)
Around the Wicket (2000)
It's Never Too Late (2001)

short stories

Bilbury Pie (1995)

on cricket

Thomas Winsden's Cricketing Almanack (1983)
Diary Of A Cricket Lover (1984)

as Edward Vernon

Practice Makes Perfect (1977)
Practise What You Preach (1978)
Getting Into Practice (1979)
Aphrodisiacs – An Owner's Manual (1983)
Aphrodisiacs – An Owner's Manual (Turbo Edition) (1984)
The Complete Guide To Life (1984)

as Marc Charbonnier

Tunnel (novel 1980)

with Alice

Alice's Diary (1989)
Alice's Adventures (1992)

with Dr Alan C Turin

No More Headaches (1981)

How To Live Longer
(And Look And Feel Younger)

Vernon Coleman

European Medical Journal

Published by the European Medical Journal, Publishing House, Trinity Place, Barnstaple, Devon EX32 9HJ, England.

Dedicated to Donna Antoinette Coleman, my Welsh Princess

ISBN: 1 898947 24 4

A catalogue record for this book is available from the British Library.

Printed by J.W. Arrowsmith Ltd., Bristol

Contents List

Preface

There is much more to life than simple good health. But good health is the foundation upon which everything else rests. Without good health none of us can enjoy life to the full.

We know more about staying healthy – and fighting disease – than at any other time in history. But finding the truth about medical matters is just as difficult as it has ever been. In some ways the explosion in research and the increased availability of medical information has made the truth even more difficult to find.

Who do you trust? How can you tell whether or not a doctor is being paid to do or say something by a drug company with a product to sell? How can you be sure that the doctor advocating a particular treatment technique is not just trying to win another patient? And how do you compare different medical and surgical techniques?

Doctors who practise as surgeons invariably claim that surgery has all the answers, whereas doctors who practise as physicians will often argue that surgery is barbaric, clumsy and dangerous and should only be used as a last resort. Who is right?

The problem with finding the truth about health matters is that doctors tend to sing the tune they have been trained to sing. If you are suffering from cancer then a surgeon will sing the praises of surgery and a radiotherapist will sing the praises of radiotherapy. But which is the right treatment for you?

It is easy to draw an analogy between finding impartial, well-informed medical advice and finding impartial, well-informed financial advice.

If you have a sum of money to invest and you ask a bond specialist to recommend a good investment he will suggest a bond. If you talk to a stockbroker he will advise that you invest directly in shares. If you talk to an insurance company man he will want to sell you an insurance policy. And if you talk to a bank manager – hoping that he will be able to guide you to the correct type of investment – the chances are that he will not know enough about what is available and feasible to be able to offer you the accurate, impartial advice that you need.

A family doctor is the medical equivalent of a bank manager. In an ideal world you would be able to ask a general practitioner to take over, guide you and offer you accurate and impartial advice about health matters.

But most family doctors are probably too busy to have the time to spare. And, to be honest, they are probably not up to date.

In the old days most patients preferred to see an older more experienced doctor because they believed that he knew more and would have balanced his medical training with a good deal of acquired wisdom and common sense. But if a doctor qualified more than five years ago then the chances are that just about everything he learned at medical school is out of date – and that everything he has learned since he left medical school has been taught to him by drug companies. Just keeping up to date is a pretty full time job these days – and most family doctors either don't have the time or aren't prepared to spend it on keeping up.

Of course, there is one big difference between seeking investment advice and seeking medical advice. If you receive poor investment advice then the worst that is likely to happen is that you will lose your money. But if you receive bad medical advice then you may lose your life.

And that brings me to the purpose of this book.

I have argued for the whole of my professional life that every individual should have the right to take control of his or her own health.

You should make the decisions about what happens to you. It is your life and only you can know what is right for you. You should not allow anyone to make vital decisions for you. Doctors make mistakes and most have a vested interest of some kind.

Obviously, if you follow this philosophy then you will need information and advice. And that is where I believe I can help you.

The book contains information and advice gathered from specialists around the world. My aim is simply to help you make better decisions about your own health and health care – and about how to live longer and stay healthier and as 'young' as possible. The final responsibility is still yours – as it should be.

This advice I give is always the advice I would take myself – or the advice I would give to someone close to me.

Although I used to be a general practitioner I no longer practise medicine and so have no allegiance to any particular branch of the profession. I can approach each subject relatively free of prejudices or preconceived notions.

And although I have grave reservations about many aspects of modern medicine I refuse to throw out the good with the bad. I believe that orthodox medicine sometimes offers the best form of treatment and that alternative medicine sometimes offers the best. I believe in a pick and mix philosophy. I am happy to take the best from any form of medicine.

Much of what you read here may surprise you. It may nòt fit comfortably with what you may have heard from the medical establishment. Remember that the medical establishment is controlled by the drug industry and that drugs are manufactured with the primary aim of making money for the companies that make them.

I am not, of course, trying to take over your doctor's job. That would be irresponsible and foolish. My aim is to help you get the best out of your doctor.

And it would be quite against my philosophy to try to give you specific advice: my aim is to help you take responsibility for your own health.

I will give you the best information and the best general advice I can. And because I believe that good health involves more than just a healthy body — it also requires a healthy mind and spirit too — this book will deal with the mind and the spirit as well as the body.

You and I may never meet. But I hope that through this book we can become good friends with a common aim: continued good health for ourselves and for those we love and care about.

Vernon Coleman 2001

Introduction

So far this week I have received details of three 'wonder' products which guarantee me perfect health and long life. Two of the distributors offer a money back refund to anyone not absolutely delighted. One of the products also promises me untold wealth, good luck at the casinos, a promotion at work, incredible energy and irresistible sexual appeal.

It is the modern way.

Read a newspaper or magazine article on ageing and you'll probably find someone recommending that the best way to live to be 100 is to eat a special extract taken from a type of seaweed collected by native virgin girls from a short stretch of New Zealand coastline. The seaweed extract will come in a beautiful package and will cost you a small fortune. If it isn't seaweed extract it will be a special, previously unheard of mineral supplement which 150-year-old peasants dig out of rocks making up the foothills of some Himalayan mountain. And if it isn't the previously unheard of mineral supplement it will be some other magical ingredient guaranteed to give long life and good health.

These sort of recommendations are immensely popular because they provide an easy, instant, painless (except for the price) solution to a problem we all want to avoid.

And we have become addicted to quick-fix solutions. Even though we may know that they won't really work we still allow ourselves to be conned by the people selling these magical remedies because we want to believe that there is an easy solution. I know intelligent, well-educated, well-informed people who regularly fall for these claims and constantly claim to be surprised and disappointed when the new 'wonder' substance they have bought turns out to be about as effective as tongue of newt and eye of toad.

Every year millions and millions of overweight people decide that they want to lose weight.

They all know that they are overweight because they have eaten too much food. By and large (with very few exceptions) that is the only way to become overweight. They know, in their hearts, that the only sure way to lose weight and stay slim is to change their eating habits permanently.

But the slimming industry doesn't get rich by selling sensible slimming advice.

It gets rich by selling miracle cures that guarantee a rapid weight loss with no effort.

Many years ago a man I knew edited a slimming magazine and I once picked up a copy of one of his magazines and thought I spotted an article I'd seen before.

'Didn't you run something like this a few months ago?' I asked him, surprised.

'Oh yes,' he replied, with disarming honesty. 'Every few months I restart the cycle.'

I stared at him. 'But don't the readers complain?'

'Oh no!' he replied. 'They never read the magazine. They buy it every month, but they don't read it. Buying the magazine is the easy bit. It shows that they're serious about losing weight. But going on a diet is the hard bit. They don't want to do that.'

'But they'll never lose weight just by buying the magazine!' I protested.

'Of course not. But these days people prefer the easy solution – even if it doesn't work.'

For years I didn't want to believe him.

But, of course, he was absolutely right. Most people do prefer simple, quick-fix solutions.

***

Just as there are no miracle pills available to help you slim rapidly, safely and permanently so there are, of course, no miracle pills available to help you live longer (or to help you stay young for the rest of your life).

But, just as there are effective ways to lose weight permanently, so there are ways to live longer. You can live longer. And you can stay young for the rest of your life.

The choice is yours.

We're all getting older. We're getting older every day. Our skin is becoming dry, flaky and not quite so soft as it was. Our hair is thinning and greying. Our reactions are slower than they were. Our joints are beginning to creak. Our hearing deteriorates. Our immune defence systems stop functioning as effectively. Bits that were firm are probably beginning to sag.

But the rate at which we age and the rate at which we appear to age are not necessarily the same thing at all.

We all know thirty year olds who look forty (or more) and we all know fifty year olds who could pass for forty (or less). If you visit an old school reunion take a good look at your contemporaries. Some will look their age. Some will look older than they are. And some will look as if they've hardly aged at all.

Whether your body looks older or younger than it really is depends upon how well you are looking after yourself. If you look after yourself (by which I mean looking after both your body and your mind) you can knock ten years (or more) off your appearance. Even more important, perhaps, you can add ten (or more) years to your prospective life expectancy. Ageing – looking and feeling older – isn't a necessary consequence of old age. You can live longer and you can live younger too.

***

Regular readers of newspapers and viewers of television programmes could be forgiven for believing that longevity is largely influenced by genetic factors.

It isn't.

Genetic influences are of little account. Your genes don't care whether you live to be 35 or 70. Your genes just want you to live long enough to procreate. Once you've reached that age the rest of your life is an irrelevance as far as your genes are concerned. There are no genes for longevity. Fewer than 10% of all cancers are genetically linked or influenced. And inheriting a cancer gene doesn't mean that you will get that particular type of cancer. It means that you have an increased risk of developing that type of cancer. There has been much talk of a breast cancer gene (BRCA-1) but there isn't really any such thing. There is no gene which causes breast cancer. There is, however, a gene which increases a woman's chances of developing cancer. Women with this gene can dramatically reduce their risk of developing breast cancer by avoiding the factors which are known to be associated with breast cancer. They should, for example, avoid becoming overweight and they should eat a low fat diet. In my view the modern 'scientific' approach (to remove the healthy breasts of women who have the breast cancer gene) is barbaric and unnecessary.

The influence that genes have on life expectation (and that influence is relatively trivial) is largely incidental. For example, there are genes which decide whether or not you have a type A (rather pushy, hard working) personality. This type of personality is an advantage early on in life. If you are pushy and hard working you will be more likely to find a mate and to be able to feed your children. As far as your genes are concerned that is a good thing. However, as you grow older so this type of personality is likely to become a burden – dramatically increasing your chances of having a heart attack. Genes only promote longevity indirectly and behaviour and lifestyle are factors which have a far greater influence on life expectation. The older you get the less effect your genes have on your health.

Having said that it is important to look at your family history and to identify the diseases which killed your ancestors. With this information you can make intelligent decisions about how you can best avoid those health problems. If you have a family history of diabetes, high blood pressure, heart disease or cancer then you may be able to dramatically increase your life expectation by doing what you can to avoid those problems.

Average life expectation could easily be 85 – or even higher – if more people took a little care with their health. But, amazingly, most people still eat too much fat, are overweight, take too little exercise, drink too much alcohol, smoke too much tobacco and do little or nothing to help themselves deal with the inevitable stresses of life in the twenty-first century.

Chapter One

How To Stay Young While Growing Old

There are a mass of misconceptions about growing old, but the commonest – and most significant – is that ageing must inevitably be associated with illness, weakness, disability and a remorseless deterioration in physical and mental health.

Accompanying this misconception is the myth that people who are classified as 'old' will need and want to spend their days sitting or lying down, and generally avoiding any sort of strenuous activity. It is probably no coincidence that accommodation for the elderly is often provided in buildings which are described as 'rest homes'.

Retirement should be a time for exploration, for freedom and for adventure. Instead it is, for most people, a time when they find themselves obliged to hand over their hard earned savings to the owner of a nursing or rest home.

Every day each of us is getting older. That is an inescapable rule of life. Two factors influence your health, your life expectancy and the rate at which your chronological age affects your ability to enjoy life.

The factor which influences your health, your susceptibility to illness, your life expectation and the rate at which you grow old (and feeble) is your lifestyle. And you can have as much control over this as you wish. If you smoke, drink too much alcohol, eat too much fatty food and spend all day sitting on the couch watching TV then you probably won't live as long and as healthy a life as you would have done if you had been a little more sensible. If you allow yourself to lie in bed all day and be waited upon, your body will become steadily weaker and weaker. The more you allow yourself to become dependant the more dependant you will become.

If you eat foods that are coated and laced with chemicals then you will become weaker and more susceptible to disease.

Heart disease, cancer and other killers become commoner as we age – but they become commoner not as a direct result of the ageing process but because of the ways in which we abuse and mistreat our bodies by (among other things) failing to exercise properly, eating poorly and exposing ourselves to unlimited amounts of stress.

The truth is that much (though obviously not all) of the disability which makes the final few decades of life so tiresome to so many people is optional. People don't choose to be ill, of course; but many do become ill and dependant because they have not chosen to be healthy. Old age is not a biological condition – and most of the symptoms which we usually associate with old age are reversible. If your lifestyle does not control your body then in the end your body will control your lifestyle.

***

Look around you and you will see evidence to support the argument that the signs of ageing are not exclusively suffered by those who have aged. Old age can occur at any age. Just what constitutes 'old' is a rather subjective issue. I know of individuals in their 80s who do not consider themselves to be 'old'. And I know men and women in their mid to late 70s who spend their time rushing around helping people whom they (with absolutely no sense of irony) describe as 'old'. As with most things in life attitude of mind is crucial.

All the changes which we usually associate with old age can occur at any age. Young people who stay in bed (either because of illness or laziness) quickly begin to display the signs normally associated with old age.

When a Swedish physiologist asked five young men to stay in bed 24 hours a day for three weeks all five suffered a dramatic drop in their aerobic capacity. The change they suffered was equivalent to almost 20 years of ageing.

Too much rest, and too little exercise, cause an enormous number of damaging changes in the body; including an increase in the proportion of body fat, a loss of body water, a reduced ability to control the body's internal temperature, a rise in blood cholesterol, a loss of calcium from the bones, a change in the way the body deals with glucose and a reduced sense of balance. In addition there are adverse effects on the senses of taste and hearing.

There is absolutely no doubt that many of the degenerative problems which we blame on chronological age are in reality a result of immobility – and can be reversed by a change in lifestyle which includes increased activity and some exercise.

Chronic, degenerative diseases (such as many instances of heart disease, diabetes and arthritis) aren't normal or natural. It is no coincidence that degenerative diseases are a largely twentieth century phenomenon – and have developed alongside the motor car, the moving pavement and the electrically-powered golf cart. Degenerative diseases are more common among people who are older because they have had more time (and more chances) to damage and misuse their bodies.

Is it any wonder that hospitals, nursing homes and rest homes are full of people who can hardly move let alone walk when, in large areas of the 'developed' world (including the whole of the US), one in two individuals are seriously overweight and one in four confess to living almost totally sedentary lives?

***

It is not possible to avoid all illness and disability, any more than it is possible to avoid old age. Ageing is an immutable force and we are mortal creatures. But it is possible to reduce your chances of showing your age – and dramatically to increase your chances of remaining active, alert and vigorous for the whole of your life.

Even if you are beginning to 'feel' your age you can take great comfort from the fact that you can regain aerobic endurance, muscular strength and the feeling of vigour and vitality which you may have thought you had lost for ever. Your age in years has very little to do with your biological age – or how old you feel.

Individuals who sit around and allow themselves to be waited upon by others will eventually become totally dependant. Their bodies will become weaker and they will lose the ability to function as independent beings. They will become fatter and their muscle mass will shrink. Immobility creates more immobility. On the other hand, those who remain determinedly as active as possible will retain their independence for as long as possible.

Many of the serious, apparently deep seated symptoms which are usually regarded as an inevitable consequence of old age can be reversed.

The philosophy to follow is a simple one: muscle strength, sexual ability, mental alertness and the ability to move around independently all depend on frequent usage. The phrase 'use it or lose it' is one which anyone who is concerned about the consequences of ageing should remember.

***

Doctors (and patients) often talk about life expectancy as though it were the only thing that mattered. Here again there are some myths which need to be exposed. The big question is: For how much of your life will you remain active and independent?

First, it is important to remember that if life expectancy is rising at all (and most doctors and drug companies would like us to believe it has risen dramatically during the last few decades) it isn't rising by very much.

Any improvement in adult life expectation which has taken place in the last century or so has been a result not of more drugs and cleverer doctors but of better sewage facilities, less overcrowding and cleaner drinking water (that one is becoming something not many of us can take for granted unless we drink filtered water or spring water).

The truth is that (as I show in the next chapter) adult life expectancy has changed very little this century (or, indeed, for many centuries). Any increase in average life span has been largely a result of lower infant mortality rates – and these have changed despite, rather than because of, doctors and drug companies.

Second, although it is something doctors never seem keen to measure, the quality of life has, for many people and many decades, been steadily going down rather than up.

Millions of people now expect their last years of life to be spent sitting in a chair or lying in bed. They expect to have to be looked after; they expect walking, dancing, cycling and sex to be memories and they expect to get winded playing anything more energetic than bridge or chess.

This is, of course, all extremely depressing because for most people the quality of life can be just as important as the quantity of life.

Most people would like their active life expectation (the number of years for which they will be able to remain self-reliant and independent) to be as close as possible to their life expectation – and they would like their personal 'disability zone' (the years for which they will be dependant on others) to be as short as possible.

***

Many doctors quite wrongly assume that weakness and frailty are inevitable consequences of ageing. This is total nonsense for which there is not a scrap of evidence. Much of the erroneous evidence used by doctors who believe that ageing must inevitably lead to dependence is a result of animal experiments.

To learn more about ageing human beings, we have to study ageing human beings. It makes no sense to try to adapt conclusions based upon animal studies or even studies of young adults.

Most people would probably list an increased susceptibility to disorders such as 'heart disease', 'stroke', 'diabetes' and so on as signs of ageing. But these are specific diseases which can happen at any age. They are not an inevitable consequence of growing old; they are not linked to ageing so much as to the changes which can complicate ageing. And you can largely control the onset and development of these changes.

***

The human body consists of two main parts: fat (or adipose tissue), which is metabolically inactive in that it just sits there and doesn't actually do anything, and the 'rest'. The 'rest' includes bones, liver, brain, heart and so on – but mostly it is made up of muscle. The 'rest' – the non-fat part of your body – is metabolically active though some of it – such as muscle – is much more active than other bits – such as bone. Muscles work all the time if you are active, and they are constantly burning up energy.

The purpose of muscle, brain and bone is pretty obvious. But the function of all the fat that is stored may seem to be something of a mystery. It is, however, merely an evolutionary hangover. The body stores fat to help keep it alive on days when there is no food to be eaten. The mechanisms for storing fat were developed a long time ago – long before the introduction of supermarkets – and are something of an anachronism in the modern 'developed' world. Fat storage is a hazardous anachronism.

Overweight is much commoner among people who are over 50 than among people who are under 50, but it isn't a direct consequence of ageing. We get fat as we get older not because our bodies are programmed to become bulkier as we hit certain chronological milestones but because, as we get older, we tend to do less exercise than we did when we were young, while at the same time we carry on eating as much as we did when we were exercising more.

One in two Americans is seriously overweight and the figures for other 'developed' countries aren't a great deal better.

The average 65-year-old man's body contains 18% fat at the age of 25 and, if he lives a sedentary life, 38% fat at the age of 65. For women the figures are considerably worse. The average 25-year-old woman's body contains 25% fat but if she lives a sedentary life then by the time she has reached 65 her body fat will be up to 43%.

The first problem with all that stored fat is that instead of simply helping to prevent starvation, stored body fat may lead to diabetes, heart disease, high blood pressure and a host of other serious health problems. Too much stored fat may dramatically shorten your life.

The second problem isn't quite so obvious, but in the long term it can be just as crucial. Since fat just lies there and doesn't burn up energy (while, in contrast, muscles work hard and do burn up energy) it stands to reason that someone whose body contains a good deal of muscle and not very much fat will burn up much more fuel than someone whose body contains a good deal of fat and not very much energy-burning muscle.

What this means is that someone whose body contains a lot of fat will have a low metabolic rate (they will burn up energy rather slowly) whereas someone with a more muscular body will have a high metabolic rate (they will burn up energy more quickly).

Someone whose body contains a lot of fat will have difficulty losing weight even if they eat very little. In contrast, someone whose body contains a lot of muscle (and not much fat) can eat huge meals without putting on weight.

***

The average individual's metabolic rate drops about 2% per decade after the age of 20. Because of this drop in the metabolic rate the average individual needs 100 calories less per day from the age of 20 onwards. After the age of 30 the calorie need drops another 100 calories. And each decade afterwards the calorie need drops by an additional 100 calories. The result is that most people need 600 calories a day less at the age of 80 than they needed at 20.

The tragedy, of course, is that most people eat more – not less – as they get older.

It is perhaps hardly surprising that unwanted weight is such a huge problem.

***

As we get older, and our bodies get fatter, we also tend to lose muscle mass. (People who maintain their weight as they age often do so because they lose muscle as they gain fat.)

Studies in the US have shown that after the age of about 20, Americans lose about 6.6 pounds (3 kilograms) of lean body mass each decade of their lives.

Between the ages of 20 and 70 we lose almost a third of our muscle cells – and the ones that are left get smaller.

Most of the muscle we lose goes not because we get older but because we don't use it. This is another example of the 'use it or lose it' philosophy I have already mentioned.

As we get older we tend to take less exercise – and the less exercise we take the more difficult we find that exercise becomes. The less we exercise the weaker we become, and the weaker we become the less we exercise. None of this has anything to do with chronological age – it is a consequence of social changes, habits and expectations.

Losing muscle is bad news for several reasons.

The first problem is, as I have already explained, that when the percentage of muscle to fat in your body drops, your metabolic rate also falls. As your metabolic rate falls so you will find that more and more of the food you eat is turned into fat – and your weight will go up. This will make it harder for you to exercise. And you will lose even more muscle. The vicious circle tightens.

The second problem is that when the amount of muscle in your body drops your aerobic capacity will also fall. Muscles consume oxygen and help keep your heart (and the rest of your cardiovascular system) working efficiently. Less muscle means a lower aerobic capacity. And your cardiovascular system will suffer.

The third problem with losing muscle is that your body won't use as much insulin. And you will be more likely to develop diabetes.

The fourth problem is that although much of the carbohydrate we eat is used up to provide us with the energy we need in order to function, the excess carbohydrate will normally be turned into glycogen and stored in the muscles where it remains as a reserve energy source.

But the less muscle you have the less glycogen your body will be able to store.

Older people who have reduced amounts of muscle will store relatively small amounts of glycogen and will, therefore, get tired easily when they exert themselves. (To make matters worse, if muscle mass is poor and excess carbohydrate cannot be stored as glycogen it will be turned into fat.)

Finally, having less muscle will also mean that your bones will become weaker (and more fragile) and your body will contain higher levels of damaging cholesterol.

Losing muscle really is bad news on a big scale.

If you are beginning to feel rather miserable by what I've written so far you can start cheering up now for numerous studies have shown that 50, 60, 70, 80 and 90 year olds can increase muscle strength and size through exercise. Age is irrelevant. Someone who exercises will gain muscle in just the same way – however old they are.

An eight week study showed that a group of male and female nursing home residents in their late 80s and 90s succeeded in increasing muscle strength and size by 10% when they exercised. Their leg muscle strength almost tripled and they were much more confident in their ability to walk than they had been before they started exercising.

It is clear that gaining new muscle – like losing old muscle – has absolutely nothing to do with how old you are.

***

Many people who are ageing badly – and who are concerned about their increasing inability to remain independent – regard losing weight as the Holy Grail that may save them from a final decade or two of incontinent indignity.

If only they can lose weight, they think, they will be able to avoid having to waste the remaining hours of their retirement years in a plastic chair, being entirely reliant upon others for every one of their basic needs.

But simply losing weight isn't enough – and won't necessarily be a help at all to anyone hoping to regain their health and fitness.

Muscle weighs more than fat and an unhealthy individual whose body contains a high percentage of fat may weigh less than a much healthier individual whose body contains a high percentage of muscle.

Losing weight through losing body fat may help you fit into clothes which are a size or two smaller but it won't help you very much if your aim is to become more active and independent. To become active and independent you will need more muscle – and simply losing weight won't help your body create more muscle.

One big problem with height weight tables is that they don't tell you how much of your body is fat. If your body is packed with muscle you could be overweight but healthy.

The other big problem with height weight tables is that they don't tell you where your body fat is stored. And the evidence shows that where your fat is stored may have a tremendous impact on your future health. (Although even if your body fat is stored in a relatively safe position it is, of course, an excellent idea to get rid of excess fat as soon as you can.)

If your fat is stored at or above waist level you are much more likely to be at risk than if your fat is stored on or below your hips.

The pear-shaped individual – with a relatively slight upper body but a relatively large bottom – is less at risk from a whole range of potentially lethal disorders (including heart disease, diabetes and stroke) than the apple-shaped individual who has his or her body fat stored above his hips.

This factor is so important that it appears that even if you are not overweight – but have a good proportion of your body fat stored above your hips – then you may be more at risk than someone who is slightly overweight but whose fat is stored at or below hip level.

So, how do you find out if your fat distribution is healthy – or hazardous? Just looking at yourself in a mirror and trying to decide whether your body shape can best be compared to an apple or a pear isn't very scientific.

So, here is a rather more objective way of doing things.

Begin by measuring your waist and your hips.

Don't suck in your tummy or breathe out when measuring your waist. And measure your hips or bottom at the largest spot.

A fabric tape measure – the sort which is commonly used by tailors and dressmakers – will do fine. It doesn't matter whether you take these measurements in inches or centimetres as long as you use the same for both measurements.

When you have taken these two measurements divide your waist measurement by your hip measurement. And check the result on this chart:

Men

Age	Low Risk	Medium Risk	High Risk	Very High Risk
20-29	<0.82	0.83 – 0.87	0.88 – 0.94	> 0.94
30-39	<0.83	0.84 – 0.90	0.91 – 0.95	> 0.96
40-49	<0.86	0.87 – 0.94	0.95 – 1.00	> 1.01
50-59	<0.87	0.88 – 0.95	0.96 – 1.00	> 1.01
60+	<0.88	0.88 – 0.97	0.98 – 1.00	> 1.01

Women

Age	Low Risk	Medium Risk	High Risk	Very High Risk
20-29	<0.72	0.73 – 0.78	0.79 – 0.81	> 0.82
30-39	<0.72	0.73 – 0.78	0.79 – 0.82	> 0.83
40-49	<0.72	0.73 – 0.78	0.79 – 0.84	> 0.85
50-59	<0.73	0.74 – 0.80	0.81 – 0.87	> 0.88
60+	<0.74	0.75 – 0.81	0.82 – 0.87	> 0.88

Men usually have a noticeably higher waist-to-hip ratio than women. On men fat is usually deposited around the waistline. Women's fat, on the other hand, is commonly collected on and around the hips and buttocks. However, when a woman deviates from the normal for her sex, she moves into a high risk category at a lower figure than would put a man into a high risk category.

***

For many years I was not enthusiastic about the value of exercise in a weight reducing programme. To get rid of a pound of fat you have to burn up 3,500 calories – and that means that a week's hard exercise programme would probably not result in the loss of a single pound of fat. (When you take into consideration the energy bars and extra food you might eat as a result of all that exercise, the value of exercise in a weight-loss programme seems to fall still further.)

But I'm now convinced that exercise does have a part to play if you are trying to lose body fat and improve the ratio of muscle to fat in your body. The best way to lose fat is through a combination of diet and exercise.

Exercise is valuable because it will help you maintain and improve your muscle mass and it will, therefore, raise your metabolic rate and make it easier for you to burn up fat.

If you try losing weight without exercising there is a danger that you will lose muscle as well as fat. That will result in a lower metabolic rate which will, in turn, make it harder for you to burn up unwanted fat.

You must, incidentally, be prepared for the fact that if you lose fat and gain muscle you may end up not losing much (if any) weight at all.

***

Losing weight and improving muscle mass and power will help you feel younger and act with more vigour. As a bonus you will probably find that as you exercise and increase your muscle mass and power you will also improve your body's aerobic capacity.

The phrase 'aerobic capacity' describes your body's ability to breathe in large amounts of oxygen (as air) and to pump and deliver large volumes of oxygen-containing blood to the various parts of your body.

Aerobic capacity normally declines with age – starting to fall at the age of around 20 in men and 30 in women. By the age of 65 our aerobic capacity is usually 30% to 40% less than it was when we were young.

There are several reasons for this decline. First, the older heart doesn't react as well to exercise. Second, it is usually smaller than it was. Third, the maximum possible heart rate drops with age too.

But the good news is that here is yet another sign of ageing that can be reversed. Your heart and general cardiovascular system probably won't change directly as a result of losing weight and gaining muscle mass but the change in your muscles will improve your aerobic capacity and the end result will be improved aerobic fitness. That is, as they say, a good thing.

***

Improving your muscle power, reducing the proportion of fat in your body and improving your aerobic capacity are by no means the only things you can do to help yourself stay young while growing old. You can also improve the way your body controls your blood sugar levels.

I have already explained that as we get older most of us take less exercise and become rather sedentary. Our bodies tend to start storing rather too much fat.

At the same time as all this is happening the tissues in our bodies appear to lose their sensitivity to insulin (the hormone which enables our bodies to metabolise the glucose in our bloodstream). This results in our tissues becoming less capable of using the sugar in our blood. And that results in the fact that even though our pancreatic glands try to increase the production of insulin our blood sugar levels tend to rise as we get older.

There aren't usually any symptoms accompanying this change but raised blood sugar levels do result in an increased chance of developing 'maturity onset diabetes'.

(Like so many other changes which are usually regarded as being associated with the ageing process these changes start at the age of about 30 years onwards. It should by now be clear that the physiological effects of ageing aren't something that just occur when we reach pensionable age. Most of the serious signs of ageing that expose us to an enhanced risk of developing degenerative diseases begin in early adulthood.)

The traditional medical approach to these raised blood sugar levels is usually to prescribe drugs to try and push the pancreas into producing more insulin. These drugs are not without their hazards and I think there is a much better way for most of us to improve the way in which our bodies deal with sugar.

(Doctors and drug companies won't tell you this sort of stuff because they are in the business of selling drugs. I make no apology for repeating the fact that, time and time again simple but effective techniques are ignored because they offer the drug industry no chance of making a profit.)

The body's gradually increasing inability to deal with sugar is, it seems, more a result of the change in the body's fat/muscle proportions than a result of an ageing, malfunctioning or inefficient pancreas.

Normally, when we eat something the muscle tissues in our bodies respond to the insulin which is produced by the cells in the pancreas glands, and then start to use the sugar in our blood. Without that triggering insulin our tissues would starve to death and our blood glucose levels would just keep rising.

As we age, however, and we lose muscle tissue and gain fat deposits, our bodies respond less and less well to the insulin which is produced.

Inactivity, a fat-rich diet and increased body fat, mean that it takes more and more insulin to stimulate the muscles and, therefore, keep the blood sugar levels under control.

To make things worse the pancreas is one of those parts of the body which does tend to work less efficiently as we age and the increased need for insulin comes at a time of life when the production of insulin is naturally slowing down.

Nevertheless, I really don't think that the use of drugs to try and kick the pancreas into working harder is the best answer to this problem.

A high fibre, low fat diet (consisting, for example, of plenty of whole grains and raw vegetables), together with regular exercise, can often lower body fat levels (thereby automatically increasing the proportion of muscle) and increase the body's sensitivity to the insulin which is being produced.

***

High blood pressure is known as the silent killer for two very good reasons: it doesn't usually produce any symptoms and it can kill.

Many doctors believe that high blood pressure is an inevitable consequence of ageing. They are wrong. Lots of people in their 70s, 80s and 90s have perfectly normal blood pressure.

High blood pressure may be inherited but in most people it is caused by a number of identified – and avoidable – lifestyle factors. Overweight, smoking, a high fat diet, stress and a lack of exercise can all contribute to a blood pressure problem. The influence of all these factors is constantly under-estimated; particularly, I'm sad to say, by a medical profession which seems determined to keep drug company profits high by insisting on pre-scribing powerful (and often potentially hazardous) drugs for the treatment of this problem, despite the fact that research has shown that these lifestyle factors are often crucially important.

(As evidence supporting the argument that lifestyle can be as signifi-cant as genetics, consider what we know about black people. Black people are unusually prone to high blood pressure but when black American men were compared with bushmen in northern Botswana it was found that the Africans didn't really begin to show signs of high blood pressure until they were in their 70s, whereas the Americans (who drank, smoke and ate too much and exercised too little) had high blood pressure in their 50s. The conclusion from this must be that a genetic predisposition can be triggered by the wrong lifestyle.)

You can probably keep your blood pressure down by eating wisely, exercising regularly, avoiding tobacco and minimising your exposure to stress.

***

Broken bones are the leading cause of accidental death in frail elderly people. A high proportion of elderly women and elderly men suffer hip fractures.

However, it is a myth that weak bones, or osteoporosis, are a normal part of the ageing process.

On the contrary, it is now clear that osteoporosis is caused by, among other things, eating the wrong sort of diet and taking too little exercise. I am constantly appalled when I hear of elderly patients being confined to bed for no very good reason. Two weeks of complete bed rest can cause the bones to lose as much calcium as would normally be lost in a year. Even when patients who are in bed cannot walk around under their own steam, they can still benefit if they are helped to get out of bed and stand on their own feet. When patients who are resting in bed are made to stand for a while every day they stop losing calcium. They don't even have to walk because the stress imposed by gravity is enough to 'persuade' the bones to retain their calcium. When you put stress on a bone it gets stronger. (Obvi-ously, some patients do have to remain in bed. But the number of patients who can't get out of bed and simply stand is very small. Talk to the doctor if he says a patient must stay in bed and ask him/her to explain why.) Oste-oporosis is not an inevitable accompaniment of ageing. It can be avoided. (See also my book *Food for Thought* published by the European Medical Journal.)

***

Some of the body's protective and healing mechanisms do deteriorate with ageing. One of the systems which tends to work less efficiently with age is the body's thermostat – the inbuilt temperature control system which, in a young, healthy body, normally keeps the internal temperature within a degree or so of 98.6 degrees Fahrenheit whatever the outside temperature might be.

When the outside temperature is hot the thermostat makes us sweat to keep cool and drink plenty of fluid to replace the fluid we lose. When the outside temperature is cold the thermostat makes us shiver to keep warm.

These mechanisms do not work as well in an elderly body – though age is not the only factor and there is no doubt that a low level of fitness and aerobic capacity damages the thermostat and makes things far worse than they otherwise would be.

The feeling of thirst is one of the vital temperature control mechanisms which does tend to deteriorate most noticeably. Older people don't feel thirsty as much or as readily as young people. This is undoubtedly the main reason why so many people in their 60s and beyond simply don't drink enough water.

I don't think there is anything you can do to improve a fading temperature control mechanism. But by making sure that you drink plenty of clean (and preferably chemical-free) water you can certainly take another step towards helping your body stay healthy.

***

Older people are far more susceptible to infection and this is largely due to the fact that their immune systems are in poor working order.

The immune system does not automatically 'fail' with age. It becomes less effective because of poor eating habits and too much stress. I explained how to keep the immune system healthy in my book *Superbody* (also published by the European Medical Journal).

***

Some things do change with age. For example, men whose fathers and grandfathers were bald will probably lose their hair as they get older. Hair loss is genetically controlled and I'm still not convinced that there is a great deal you can do to stop it.

On the other hand there is no real reason why the skin should suffer as much as it often does. Regular and generous use of a plain moisturising cream – and not spending too much time in the sun – can help the skin stay supple, wrinkle free and young looking.

***

At regular intervals doctors, anthropologists and journalists discover groups of people in various parts of the 'undeveloped' world who seem to have found the secret of long life. Some of these discoveries are probably falsely based. Birth records aren't always reliable in distant country areas. But whatever the truth may be about some of the astonishing longevity claims which have been made in recent years one thing is clear: there are a number of similarities between the people in different parts of the world who succeed in living long and healthy lives:

- ◆ Obesity is uncommon.
- ◆ Diets are low in animal fats.
- ◆ Consumption of tobacco and alcohol is low.
- ◆ Retirement is unknown and the elderly retain their social status and the respect of the young.
- ◆ Daily physical activity is commonplace.
- ◆ Outside (or 'toxic') stress is minimal.

If you look down this list and then think about how we run our lives it is difficult to escape the conclusion that we seem to be doing our very best to ensure that we age rapidly and spend our final years dependant upon others for virtually everything we need.

In our modern 'developed' world millions of people in their 40s and beyond are overweight; overfed (with all the wrong sorts of highly refined high fat foods); polluted and poisoned by the air they breathe, the water they drink, the food they eat and the drugs they are encouraged to swallow; exposed to virtually unlimited quantities of 'toxic' stress, constantly frustrated and hassled and seriously undervalued by society at large.

***

You can stay young while growing old. And the final proof that it is possible to stay young while growing old comes from research done on 7,000 residents of Alameda County, California.

Investigators there showed that 70 year olds who didn't smoke, who kept their weight within 20% of the recommended level for their age; who drank moderate amounts of alcohol (some alcohol is better for you than no alcohol – and obviously better than too much); who took moderate exercise three times a week; who slept seven or eight hours a night and who ate regularly (including at breakfast time) were as healthy as people in their late 30s and early 40s who practised only half of these simple rules. The researchers showed that men who followed these simple guidelines lived, on average, eleven years longer than men who didn't while women lived, on average, an extra seven years.

And if you really want to improve your chances of staying healthy and active and independent until the end of your life you should remember that maintaining a useful and satisfying role in the world is one of the most crucial keys to staying young while growing old. ✳

Chapter Two

Plan Now To Avoid An Inevitable Health Crisis

Back in 1988, in my book *The Health Scandal*, I forecast that by the year 2020 one third of the population in the developed world would be over the age of 65 and that in every home where there were two healthy parents and two healthy children there would be four disabled or dependent individuals needing constant care.

I predicted that diseases such as diabetes (which is genetically transmitted) and blindness (which is ten times as common among the over 65s and thirty times as common among the over 75s) would be as common as indigestion and hay fever are today, that unemployment would be common, that stress-related diseases would be endemic and that developed countries around the world would face bankruptcy as they struggled to find the cash to pay pensions, sick pay and unemployment benefits.

I forecast that, tragically and unfairly, resentment, bitterness and anger would divide the young and the old, the able bodied and the dependent, the employed and the unemployed; and that there would, within 20 years of the start of the twenty-first century, be anarchy, despair and civil war with ghettoes of elderly and disabled citizens abandoned to care for themselves.

For years those who have forecast the end of the human race have talked of nuclear war, starvation in the third world and pollution as being the major threats to our survival. But back in 1988 I argued that the decline I predicted for the year 2020 would be triggered not by any of these forces but by much simpler and entirely predictable developments.

All the evidence I have seen in the years since I made those predictions convinces me that I was right. We are heading for a medical and social catastrophe. And every day that goes by makes that catastrophe increasingly inevitable. Everyone will suffer: today's elderly, tomorrow's elderly and tomorrow's young too.

When I first published this forecast the medical and political establishments refused to take my warning seriously. I was dismissed as a scaremonger. No one would broadcast the TV series I wanted to make and the book I wrote about the whole issue (called *The Health Scandal*) was studiously ignored. Even though I personally bought around two thousand copies of the book and subsequently sent copies to every Member of Parliament in Britain, most leading journalists, many doctors and hundreds of public libraries the whole issue remained largely undiscussed.

Now, at last, some sections of the media have begun to recognise that we are truly facing a colossal problem – and that the growing size of our elderly and disabled populations will pose enormous problems to our society. But neither politicians nor commentators have yet stumbled on the true background explanation for what is happening – and nor have they offered any practical advice on how you can best protect yourself against the problems which are coming.

When I wrote *The Health Scandal* I estimated that by 2020 we would have reached the position where more than half the population would be 'dependant' – either through age or disability.

It now looks as if my calculations were accurate. If anything they were rather conservative. There seems to me to be little doubt that in the next thirty years age will have a far more divisive effect on our society than race, sex or class have ever had. By 2020 the disabled and incapable will outnumber the healthy and able bodied.

In developed countries total populations are increasing very slowly, but the ageing populations are increasing at a dramatic rate. For example, during one recent decade the total population of Britain increased by less than 1%. But in the same period the pensionable population rose by 10%. In many westernised nations one person in five is already a pensioner.

By the year 2020 a third of the population in most developed countries will be pensioners.

Several things make this explosion in the size of the elderly population particularly significant.

First, there is the fact that among older populations there is a higher proportion of disabled and dependent individuals. The incidence of chronic disease rises rapidly among older age groups. (Though, as I have already shown, this is largely because people fail to look after themselves effectively.)

- ♦ Among 16 to 44 year olds 20% of the population suffer from chronic illness.

- Among 45 to 64 year olds 40% of the population suffer from chronic illness.
- Among 65 to 74 year olds 50% of the population suffer from chronic illness.
- And among people aged 75 or over 65% of the population suffer from chronic, long term illness.

Consider strokes: already half the beds in British National Health Service hospitals are occupied by patients suffering from some sort of stroke. Stroke patients generally need to stay in hospital for long periods of time and they need intensive nursing care.

Or consider diabetes. Since diabetes is a hereditary disease the incidence of this problem is increasing rapidly. The increase in the number of elderly people alive in our society merely exacerbates the problem. The incidence of diabetes is doubling every decade. In 1984 just 2% of the population in the average sort of developed, westernised country was diabetic. If the increase continues at the same rate then by the year 2020 one in four people will be diabetic. Many cases of diabetes can be avoided or controlled by diet but too often the orthodox approach is to wait until symptoms develop and then use drugs to tackle the problem.

There is also ample evidence to show that mental disease is on the increase. The number of patients with mental illness needing to be admitted to hospital is rising by 10% every decade. Today, 25% of the population will, at some stage in their lives, suffer from mental illness, often severe enough to warrant admission to a mental hospital.

One side effect of all this will be that more and more hospital beds will be blocked and unavailable for emergencies. All this will inevitably mean that waiting lists for non-urgent surgery will get longer and longer, and the number of people in our community suffering from disabling and untreated problems such as arthritic hips will grow even faster. The steady increase in our elderly population will mean that the quality of health care will steadily deteriorate.

The second reason why the explosion in the size of the elderly population is dangerous is that the number of young people is falling. And the result is that in the future a smaller and smaller working population will have to support a larger and larger dependent population.

That takes us neatly into the third reason why the explosion in the size of our over 60 population is likely to produce real problems: money.

Most workers who are currently paying pension contributions assume that the money they are paying will be invested and repaid to them when they reach pensionable age. But that is not the case. The pension contributions paid by today's workers are used to pay the pensions of yesterday's workers – today's pensioners. If pension programmes were being organised by private individuals they would be described as pyramid or Ponzi schemes and the organisers would be in prison.

The pensions that today's workers will receive when they retire will be paid by the contributions made by tomorrow's workers. But the working population is getting smaller and smaller. And the retired population is getting bigger and bigger.

You don't have to be a genius to see the disaster we are heading for.

This is, without a doubt, one of the biggest problems our society must face. It is something I've been writing about – and warning about – for over a decade, but our politicians still don't seem to have noticed it and very few members of the public seem to understand it.

The easy, and often voiced, explanation for both the increase in the size of the developed world's elderly population and the increase in the number of disabled and financially dependent individuals is that modern medical miracles, produced by the medical profession and the pharmaceutical industry, have produced the change by enabling people to live longer.

Doctors and drug companies have for some time excused their errors, and successfully distracted attention away from their incompetence, by arguing that their efforts have resulted in a consistent and impressive improvement in life expectancy during the last century or so. The increasing size of our elderly (and disabled) population is, say the industry's supporters, a direct consequence of medical progress.

The truth, however, is rather different. The medical profession and the drug companies are guilty of a confidence trick of gargantuan proportions.

The fact is that during the last century doctors and drug companies have become louder, more aggressive, a good deal richer and far more powerful, but life expectancy has hardly changed.

Improved sanitation facilities have meant that the number of babies dying – and the number of women dying in childbirth – have fallen dramatically, but for adults life expectation has not been rising.

To prove my point I arbitrarily selected a list of 111 famous individuals – all of whom lived and died before the start of this century. I then checked to see how old these individuals were when they died. I'm printing the list below because it illustrates the point I'm making – and it is an important point. The results prove my argument: life expectation (now between 70 and 75 years in developed countries) has not risen appreciably during the last century. You may find it illuminating to think of any other individuals who died before the start of this century – and to then check up to see how old they were when they died.

Andersen, Hans Christian. Died 1875 aged 70.

Aristotle. Died 322 BC aged 62.

Attila the Hun. Died in 453 BC aged 47.

Audubon, John. Died in 1851 aged 66.

Augustine, St Aurelius. Died in 430 aged 76.

Bach, JS. Died in 1750 aged 65.

Beethoven, Ludwig van. Died in 1827 aged 57.

Bentham, Jeremy. Died in 1832 aged 84.

Berlioz, Hector. Died in 1869 aged 66.

Bernini, Gian. Died in 1680 aged 82.

Bizet, Georges. Died in 1875 aged 37.

Blackmore RD. Died 1900 aged 75.

Blake, William. Died 1827 aged 70.

Botticelli, Sandro. Died in 1510 aged 66.

Brahms, Johannes. Died in 1833 aged 63.

Browning, Robert. Died 1889 aged 77.

Bruckner, Anton. Died 1896 aged 72.

Brummell, Beau. Died in 1840 aged 61.

Brunelleschi, Filippo. Died 1446 aged 69.

Canaletto. Died 1768 aged 71.

Cardigan, James , 7th Earl of. Died 1868 aged 71.

Carroll, Lewis. Died 1898 aged 66.

Casanova, Giovanni. Died 1798 aged 73.

Catherine the Great. Died in 1796 aged 67.

Charlemagne, (Charles the Great). Died 814 aged 67.

Charles 11. Died 1685 aged 55.

Chaucer, Geoffrey. Died in 1400 aged 60.

Coleridge, Samuel Taylor. Died 1834 aged 62.

Confucius. Died 479 BC aged 72.

Constable, John. Died in 1837 aged 60.

Copernicus, Nicolaus. Died in 1543 aged 70.

da Vinci, Leonardo. Died 1519 aged 67.

Daimler, Gottlieb. Died in 1900 aged 66.

Darwin, Charles. Died in 1882 aged 73.

de Cervantes, Miguel. Died in 1616 aged 69.

de Sade, Marquis. Died in 1814 aged 74.

Defoe, Daniel. Died in 1731 aged 71.

Dickens, Charles. Died in 1870 aged 58.

Disraeli, Benjamin. Died in 1881 aged 76.

Dostoyevsky, Fyodor. Died 1881 aged 60.

Dryden, John. Died 1700 aged 69.

Dumas, Alexandre. Died 1870 aged 68.

Eliot, George. (Marian Evans) Died 1880 aged 61.

Elizabeth 1. Died in 1603 aged 70.

Emerson, Ralph Waldo. Died 1882 aged 79.

Engels, Friedrich. Died 1895 aged 75.

Epicurus. Died 271 BC aged 70.

Euripides. Died in 406 BC aged 78.

Francis of Assisi. Died 1226 aged 45.

Franklin, Benjamin. Died 1790 aged 84.

Galilei, Galileo. Died 1642 aged 78.

Garibaldi, Giuseppe. Died 1882 aged 75.

George 111. Died in 1820 aged 81.

Gladstone, William. Died in 1898 aged 88.

Goethe, Johann Wolfgang von. Died 1832 aged 83.

Gounod, Charles. Died 1883 aged 65.

Greco, El. Died 1614 aged 73.

Grimm, Wilhelm. Died 1859 aged 73.

Grimm, Jacob. Died 1863 aged 78.

Handel, George. Died 1759 aged 74.

Hansard, Luke. Died 1828 aged 76.

Haydn, Franz Joseph. Died in 1809 aged 77.

Henry V111. Died in 1547 aged 56.

Herod, the Great. Died 4BC aged 70.

Hippocrates. Died in 377 BC aged 83.

Hobbes, Thomas. Died 1679 aged 91.

Hogarth, William. Died in 1764 aged 67.

Humboldt, Alexander. Died 1859 aged 90.

Johnson, Samuel. Died in 1784 aged 75.

Jones, Inigo. Died 1652 aged 79.

Kant, Immanuel. Died 1804 aged 80.

Khan, Ghengis. Died in 1227 aged 65.

Khayyam, Omar. Died in 1123 aged 73.

Kublai Khan. Died 1294 aged 80.

Liszt, Franz. Died 1886 aged 75.

Longfellow, Henry Wadsworth. Died 1882 aged 75.

Macintosh, Charles. Died 1843 aged 77.

Marx, Karl. Died 1883 aged 65.

Michelangelo. Died in 1564 aged 89.

Milton, John. Died 1674 aged 66.

Montefiore, Sir Moses. Died 1885 aged 101.

Monteverdi, Claudio. Died 1643 aged 76.

Mozart, Wolfgang Amadeus. Died in 1791 aged 35.

Nash, John. Died 1835 aged 83.

Newton, Isaac. Died in 1727 aged 84.

Nobel, Alfred. Died in 1896 aged 63.

Nostradamus. Died 1566 aged 63.

Offenbach, Jacques. Died 1880 aged 61.

Palladio. Died 1580 aged 72.

Pepys, Samuel. Died 1703 aged 70.

Plato. Died c.348 BC aged 80.

Polo, Marco. Died 1324 aged 70.

Rousseau, Jean Jacques. Died 1778 aged 66.

Ruskin, John. Died in 1900 aged 80.

Sandwich, 4th Earl of. Died 1792 aged 74.

Shakespeare, William. Died in 1616 aged 52.

Sophocles. Died in 406 BC aged 90.

Stowe, Harriet Beecher. Died in 1896 aged 85.

Stradivari, Antonio. Died in 1737 aged 93.

Tennyson, Lord Alfred. Died 1892 aged 83.

Thackeray, William Makepeace. Died 1863 aged 52.

Titian. Died in 1576 aged 99.

Turner, Joseph. Died in 1851 aged 76.

Victor Hugo. Died 1885 aged 83.

Voltaire, Francois. Died 1778 aged 84.

Washington, George. Died in 1799 aged 67.

Watt, James. Died in 1819 aged 83.

Wesley, John. Died in 1791 aged 87.

Whitman, Walt. Died 1892 aged 73.

Wordsworth, William. Died 1850 aged 80.

Wren, Christopher. Died in 1723 aged 90.

There are 111 names on this list. The average age at death was: 72.39 years. And, on average, it is 433 years since each of these individuals died.

The conclusion is simple: despite all the expensive razzmatazz of modern medicine life expectation has simply not increased in the last century or so. The biblical promise of three score years and ten has been fairly steady for centuries.

There are two reasons for the crisis we now face.

First there has, for many decades, been a steady reduction in the number of children being born in the developed world. Terrified by what was originally described as the birth explosion time bomb, millions of couples decided to limit their families – or not to have children at all. The introduction of the contraceptive pill and of sterilisation techniques for both men and women made this easy. (In contrast this has definitely not been the case in the developing world and the global political consequences are far reaching. In Muslim countries birth rates are extremely high and the average age in those populations is inevitably much younger. A society which is predominantly composed of young, healthy individuals obviously has a very different outlook to a society which is dominated by older, often unhealthy individuals. The future is Muslim. Our ageing, western, largely Christian society has very little future.)

As the number of elderly people as a percentage of the overall population has been steadily increasing so the incidence of disability among the elderly has been increasing steadily too. Today's elderly are nowhere near as fit as their ancestors were. Our fat and toxin rich diet is just one factor which has led to a steady increase in the incidence of cancer, obesity, heart disease, arthritis and many other causes of long term disability. Mental illness such as chronic anxiety and depression, caused by the unavoidable 'toxic stresses' created by the structured society in which we live (and which I described in detail in my book *How to Overcome Toxic Stress* published by the European Medical Journal) are now endemic – as are the myriad illnesses caused by the powerful drugs frequently prescribed by doctors with such carelessness.

When I wrote about this issue in a newspaper column I was swamped with letters of protest from people over the age of 60 who seemed to think that by daring to mention the existence of this problem I was in some way publishing an attack on the elderly. Many of the responses seemed to consist of hysterical abuse rather than anything else. I was not, of course, attacking the elderly, the disabled or anyone else. I was simply trying to draw attention to the problem in the hope that those in the position to do something about it might act. Most of those reading my warning completely missed the point and it is, indeed, the absence of any widespread public interest in this colossal problem which convinces me that the future is a gloomy one.

Without public interest I certainly don't think that politicians anywhere are likely to act quickly if at all. Politicians everywhere tend to think in four or five year terms at the most. They are concerned only with the now – rather than with the future – because what happens now decides whether or not they get re-elected. And professional politicians care about nothing as much as they care about political power.

Nevertheless, it is now to a large extent too late. Whether the politicians ever act or not this problem exists and it is going to affect all our lives in a very real and dramatic way. The incidence of illness and disability is going to rise and rise and the availability of public resources is going to fall and fall.

If you are currently over the age of 35 then the chances are that by the time you reach the sort of age at which you might hope to retire, you will discover that any publicly funded pension you might receive will either be very small, or non-existent, and the availability of sheltered or nursing home accommodation will be extremely limited.

If you are currently under the age of 35 then you are going to have to pay a steadily increasing percentage of your earnings in income tax and national insurance deductions. You can safely ignore anything politicians say about cutting taxes. The fact is that taxes are probably never going to be lower than they are at the moment. The young are, I suppose, in the very worst position of all. Throughout their working lives they are going to have to struggle to pay towards the care of a relatively larger and larger elderly population. When they themselves reach retirement age they will be in even bigger trouble for they will probably not have been able to save anything to look after themselves.

This is a threat no one can escape. The problem isn't going to go away and this isn't a threat that you can avoid simply by moving into a nuclear bunker in the garden for a few weeks or months.

✳   My first piece of advice is that you should do everything you can to ensure that you stay as healthy as possible in the future. Do not rely on being able to ask for or even obtain skilled and reliable medical help. The quality of health care has been sliding steadily for decades and the quantity of available care has also been diminishing. Obtaining health care is likely to be increasingly difficult and expensive. To preserve your health you must carefully watch what you eat, lose any excess weight and avoid tobacco smoke (taken directly or indirectly) whenever possible. The biggest killers (and disablers) in the developed world (cancer, heart disease and stroke) are strongly related to lifestyle. You can dramatically – and fairly easily – reduce your chances of suffering from any of these three big killers by watching what you eat, by taking modest, regular exercise (such as walking) and by increasing your resistance to, and reducing your exposure to, unwanted stress. By keeping your weight under control you will minimise your chances of developing diabetes or arthritis – two disorders which cause much immobility and disablement. ✳

Second, you must make whatever financial arrangements you can to ensure that you can afford to buy whatever professional help you may need in the future. I suggest that you do not rely on state funded schemes. Nor am I enthusiastic about privately funded health insurance schemes. I have never been a fan of private health insurance. Bureaucratic overheads mean that the premiums are often high. In addition the exclusion clauses are frequently wide ranging. There is also the problem that some private insurers won't pay for alternative therapies – even when those therapies might be safer, cheaper and more effective than orthodox therapies. If you want to buy some insurance then my own preference is for an ordinary sickness policy which simply pays out cash when you can't work. But I would supplement that, and plan for the future, simply by investing the money I would have paid for private health insurance and keeping it as a 'private' and 'personal' health nest egg. Think how much you could save in a few years by investing the sort of money private health insurers require in premiums.

Third, I think it is probably sensible to plan to spend the final third of your life in a fairly self-contained environment – and well within your means. Financially, there are hard times ahead for those who do not work. State pensions, already small, are likely to become increasingly derisory. I have absolutely no desire to offer a scary scenario for the future but I believe that all the evidence suggests that our society is going to be increasingly violent. Theft and muggings are going to become commoner and commoner. It is also likely to become increasingly difficult to find electricians, plumbers, carpenters, decorators and other tradesmen.

Fourth, learn as much as you can about how to look after yourself. Most illnesses can be safely and effectively treated without a doctor (or, indeed, an alternative health care practitioner).

You should also be constantly aware that the sad and tragic truth is that many of the chronically disabling illnesses of the twentieth century are actually caused by drug therapy.

For example, I wonder how many people know that tinnitus – that desperately depressing constant ringing of the ears which causes so much distress and ruins so many lives – is frequently a side effect of anti-depressant therapy? A reader who was put on anti-depressants and who subsequently complained of tinnitus was assured by at least six highly qualified experts that her tinnitus could not possibly have been caused by the drug she was taking. Because the tinnitus was making her more depressed they increased the dose of the drug. The tinnitus got worse. The experts seemed surprised that when she stopped the drug the tinnitus went away and the depression lifted.

Most doctors prescribe far too many different drugs and as a result they have no idea what side effects are associated with the drugs they are handing out. You should remember Coleman's First Law of Modern Medicine: 'If you develop new symptoms while being treated for any medical condition the chances are that the new symptoms are caused by the treatment you are receiving.' At least one in six patients in hospital are there because they have been made ill by doctors. The reason is simple. Few doctors know Coleman's First Law of Modern Medicine. You should never forget it. It will be a vital weapon in your armoury in the years ahead.

Chapter Three

Why You Shouldn't Trust Your Doctor

If you're going to survive to a good age – and stay healthy and young – then you need to know something about doctors. Many people are prepared to put all their trust in doctors. That, I intend to show, can be a dangerous mistake. Doctors now do more harm than good. They can – and do – save lives. But they kill a lot of people too.

The incidence of doctor-induced illness is now epidemic throughout the Western world. At any one time at least one in six patients are in hospital because of some side effect of their medication. There's now even a name for an illness caused by doctors – such illnesses are known as iatrogenic illness – and in most Western countries this problem is as big a cause of serious illness and death as are cancer or heart disease.

There is nothing new in the fact that doctors kill people. Doctors have always made mistakes and there have always been patients who have died as a result of medical ignorance or incompetence.

But, since we now spend more on health care than ever before, and since the medical profession is apparently more scientific and better equipped than ever before, there is a savage irony in the fact that we have now reached the point where, on balance, well-meaning doctors in general practice and highly trained, well-equipped specialists working in hospitals do more harm than good.

The epidemic of iatrogenic disease which has always scarred medical practice has been steadily getting worse and today most of us would, most of the time, be better off without a medical profession.

Most developed countries now spend around 8% of their gross national products on health care (the Americans spend considerably more – around 14%) but through a mixture of ignorance, incompetence, prejudice, dishonesty, laziness, paternalism and misplaced trust doctors are killing more people than they are saving and they are causing more illness and more discomfort than they are alleviating.

Most developed countries now spend around 1% of their annual income on prescription drugs, and doctors have more knowledge and greater access to powerful treatments than ever before, but there has probably never been another time in history when doctors have done more harm than they do today.

When the medical profession, together with the pharmaceutical industry, claims that it is the advances in medicine which are responsible for the fact that life expectancy figures have risen in the last one hundred years or so they are wrong.

Any improvement in life expectancy which has occurred in the last hundred years is not related to developments in the medical profession, or to the growth of the international drug industry; but the increase in iatrogenesis is related to both these factors.

Whichever facts you look at they seem to support my contention that although doctors may do a limited amount of good they do a great deal more harm.

***

If doctors really did help people stay alive then you might expect to find that the countries which had the most doctors would have the best life expectation figures. But that isn't the case at all.

Even more startling, perhaps, is the evidence of what happens when doctors betray their principles, embrace mammon, go on strike and leave patients to cope without professional medical help.

You might imagine that without doctors people would be dying like flies in autumn. Not a bit of it. When doctors in Israel went on strike for a month admissions to hospital dropped by 85% with only the most urgent cases being admitted, but despite this the death rate in Israel dropped by 50% – the largest drop since the previous doctors' strike twenty years earlier – to its lowest ever recorded level. Much the same thing has happened wherever doctors have gone on strike. In Bogota, Colombia doctors went on strike for 52 days and there was a 35% fall in the mortality rate. In Los Angeles a doctors' strike resulted in an 18% reduction in the death rate. During the strike there were 60% fewer operations in 17 major hospitals. At the end of the strike the death rate went back up to normal.

I am told that when hospitals and clinics were closed down by terrorists in Sri Lanka the Registrar General reported that the number of reported deaths had fallen.

Whatever statistics are consulted, whatever evidence is examined, the conclusion has to be the same. Doctors are a hazard rather than an asset to any community. In Britain the death rate of working men over 50 was higher in the 1970s than it was in the 1930s. The British were never healthier than they were during the Second World War.

Figures published by the United States Bureau of Census show that 33% of people born in 1907 could expect to live to the age of 75 whereas 33% of the people born in 1977 could expect to live to the age of 80. Remove the improvements produced by better living conditions, cleaner water supplies, and the reduction in deaths during or just after childbirth and it becomes clear that doctors, drug companies and hospitals cannot possibly have had any useful effect on life expectancy. Indeed, the figures show that there has been an increase in mortality rates among the middle aged and an increase in the incidence of disabling disorders such as diabetes and arthritis. The incidence of diabetes, for example, is now reported to be doubling every ten years and the incidence of serious heart disease among young men is increasing rapidly. Today, death rates from heart disease among adults are 50 times higher than they were a century ago.

***

Drugs are one of the biggest problems. Not heroin, cannabis or cocaine. Prescription drugs. If drugs were only ever prescribed sensibly, and when they were likely to interfere with a potentially life threatening disease, then the risks associated with their use would be acceptable. But all the evidence shows that doctors do not understand the hazards associated with the drugs they use and frequently prescribe inappropriately and excessively. Many of the deaths associated with drug use are caused by drugs which did not need to be taken.

Patients are given the wrong drug.

Or they are given the wrong dose of the right drug.

Or they are given the right drug by the wrong route (for example, a drug that should be injected into a muscle may be injected directly into the bloodstream).

Experts believe that there is an error roughly one in every eight times when a hospital patient is given a drug.

Since an ordinary hospital patient may receive a dozen different drugs – at different times of the day – the opportunities for error are colossal.

In a 300 bed hospital there may be between 300 and 400 medication errors every day.

Some of those errors will result in mild discomfort.

Some will result in death.

The best example of the modern tendency to over-prescribe probably lies in the way that antibiotics are used.

One in six prescriptions is for an antibiotic and there are at least 100 preparations available for doctors to choose from. When antibiotics – drugs

45

such as penicillin – were first introduced in the 1930s they gave doctors a chance to kill the bacteria causing infections.

Various independent experts who have studied the use of antibiotics claim that between 50 – 90% of the prescriptions written for antibiotics are unnecessary. To a certain extent doctors over-prescribe because they like to do something when faced with a patient – and prescribing a drug is virtually the only thing most of them can do. Also, to some extent prescribing a drug is a defence against any possible future charge of negligence (on the basis that if the patient dies it is better to have done something than to have done nothing). But the main reason for the over-prescribing of antibiotics is, without doubt, the fact that doctors are under the influence of the drug companies. The makers of the antibiotics want their drugs prescribed in vast quantities. It makes no difference to them whether or not the prescriptions are necessary.

The over-prescribing of antibiotics would not matter too much if these drugs were harmless and if there were no other hazards associated with their use. But antibiotics are certainly not harmless. The unnecessary and excessive use of antibiotics causes allergy reactions, side effects and a huge variety of serious complications – including the ultimate complication: death. There is also the very real hazard that by overusing antibiotics doctors are enabling bacteria to develop immunity to these potentially life-saving drugs. There is now no doubt that many of our most useful drugs have been devalued by overuse and are no longer effective.

To all this must be added the damage done by vaccines. I dealt with this problem at length in my book *Superbody*.

***

It is now widely accepted that at least 40% of all the people who are given prescription medicines to take will suffer uncomfortable, hazardous or potentially lethal side effects.

I say 'at least' because, for a variety of reasons, the vast majority of doctors never admit that their patients ever suffer any side effects. In Britain, for example, five out of six doctors have never reported any drug side effects to the authorities – authorities who admit that they receive information on no more than 10% – 15% of even the most serious adverse drug reactions occurring in patients. In other words they admit that they never hear about at least 85% – 90% of all dangerous drug reactions. Astonishingly, it is even accepted that some doctors will withhold reports of serious adverse reactions, and keep their suspicions to themselves, in the hope that they may later be able to win fame by publishing their findings in a journal or revealing their discovery to a newspaper or magazine.

Patients who take drugs are taking a risk; they are often taking part in a massive experiment and by taking a medicine may become worse off than if they had done nothing. To make things worse no one knows exactly how big the risks are when a particular drug is taken. All drugs are potential poisons that may heal or may kill.

The medical profession, the drug industry and the regulatory bodies all accept that the hazards of using any drug will only be known when the drug has been given to large numbers of patients for a considerable period of time.

***

One of the major reasons for the disastrously high incidence of problems associated with drug use is the fact that the initial clinical trials, performed before a drug is made available for all general practitioners to prescribe for their patients, rarely involve more than a few thousand patients at most. Some initial trials may involve no more than half a dozen patients.

However, it is now well known that severe problems often do not appear either until at least 50,000 patients have taken a drug or until patients have used a drug for many months or even years. Because of this a huge death toll can build up over the years. Drug control authorities admit that when a new drug is launched no one really knows what will happen or what side effects will be identified.

Doctors and drug companies are, it seems, using the public in a constant, ongoing, mass testing programme. And the frightening truth is that far more people are killed as a result of prescription drugs (including vaccines) than are killed as a result of using illegal drugs such as heroin or cocaine.

***

It is not only by prescribing drugs or vaccines that doctors do harm. There is plenty of evidence to show that patients are at risk in other ways.

At least 1 in 10 of all hospital patients will pick up an infection in hospital – mostly urinary tract, chest or wound infections, and mostly caused by doctors and nurses failing to wash their hands often enough.

Since Ignaz Philipp Semmelweiss first demonstrated (in the mid-19th century) that deaths in the delivery room were caused by dirty hands every child has been taught the importance of basic personal hygiene. Sadly, the message does not seem to have got through to the medical and nursing professions.

One study showed that nurses washed their hands only once every three times after cleaning around a patient's catheter.

Another study at a major hospital showed that hand washing by staff was well below recommended levels.

A study of doctors' habits showed that two out of three anaesthetists failed to wash their hands before treating a new patient (even though anaesthetists frequently perform venepuncture surgery) while one in three surgeons did not wash their arms properly before an operation.

At least one-third of all hospital infections are caused by dirty hands. And up to 1 in 10 patients in hospital acquire an infection.

The cost in simple financial terms is colossal. Treating hospital-contracted infections uses up around 15% of the hospital budget in the UK, and adds around a week to each patient's hospital stay. It is hardly surprising that waiting lists get longer and longer.

The cost in human terms is incalculable: tens of thousands of patients die because of bugs they've caught from doctors, nurses, other staff or contaminated equipment.

These aren't statistics: they are people. Real people. Every one of those unnecessary deaths is someone's wife, husband, mother, father, son, daughter, uncle, aunt, friend or neighbour.

Most of those patients die because doctors and nurses can't be bothered to wash their hands properly, or because operating theatres aren't properly cleaned between operations.

The medical answer is – surprise, surprise – often to prescribe antibiotics – a third of hospital patients end up taking them. The result is that bugs are becoming immune. And antibiotics often don't work. It takes 50 times as much penicillin to treat an infection today as it required thirty years ago.

It is hardly surprising that people who stay at home to be treated – or who go home quickly after day-case or short-stay surgery – usually get better much quicker than people who need long-stay treatment and who have to go into hospital.

***

Surgery can be pretty dangerous too.

And the danger is even more alarming when you realise that at least a quarter of operations performed are unnecessary.

For some types of surgery – heart surgery, tonsillectomies, circumcisions, Caesarean sections for pregnant women and hysterectomies, for example – the percentage of unnecessary operations is almost certainly much higher.

Some experts argue that three quarters of some types of operation are probably unnecessary.

Operations are done unnecessarily for a huge variety of reasons.

Some – particularly those performed on private patients – may be done because the surgeon needs the cash. Some patients are put down for surgery in order to keep waiting lists long – so that more patients are prepared to pay for private treatment. And some unnecessary operations are done because it's easier to cut open a patient than it is to think about alternatives.

And it isn't just a problem because of the unnecessary pain and discomfort that patients have to put up with.

At least 1% of patients who undergo surgery dies.

One in every hundred patients who goes into hospital for an operation does not walk out again afterwards.

Of course, some patients are very ill when they are wheeled into the operating theatre.

And some patients would have died anyway without surgery.

But many patients are perfectly healthy when they are taken into the operating theatre. They are having surgery because they have been persuaded by doctors that it is necessary, or that it will in some way improve the quality of their lives.

***

When doctors from the Harvard School of Public Health studied what happened to more than 30,000 patients admitted to acute care hospitals in New York, they found that nearly 4% of them suffered unintended injuries in the course of their treatment and that 14% of those patients died of their injuries. This survey concluded that nearly 200,000 people die each year in America as a result of medical accidents. This means that more than four times as many people die from injuries caused by doctors as die in road accidents. The real figure is probably considerably higher than this and there can be little doubt that many of the injuries and deaths are caused by simple, straightforward incompetence rather than bad luck or unforeseen complications.

Coronary bypass operations are immensely popular among heart surgeons (and extremely profitable) but a major study conducted in Europe showed that many patients who don't have surgery live longer than those who do. When one researcher studied 300 patients who'd had bypass operations at several hospitals in California he concluded that 14% of the patients would have thrived as well without surgery while another 30% were borderline. Around 50% of lower back disc operations and up to 70% of hysterectomies are probably unnecessary. In America the death toll from unnecessary surgery alone has been estimated to be as high as 80,000 patients per year.

***

Most people now recognise that powerful, modern medical treatments – such as drugs and surgery – can be dangerous.

Fewer people realise that even the tests doctors do before they treat a patient can often be just as dangerous.

This would not matter so much if all the tests doctors did were essential.

But astonishing and startling evidence now shows that the X-rays, blood tests and other investigations which doctors order are not just sometimes lethal but are frequently unnecessary. Many tests are wildly inaccurate and dangerously misleading as well.

Here are just some of the frightening facts that I can reveal about medical investigations:

- X-rays are the third biggest cause of cancer (after cigarette smoking and eating meat and fatty food).
- Tests often wrongly show up disease in healthy individuals. Those patients are then subjected to surgery and drug therapy which they do not need.
- Tests – which patients and doctors seem to trust too much – often wrongly say that a patient is healthy.
- About two thirds of all medical tests are worthless and of no help to the patient.
- Patients routinely admitted to hospital are often subjected to 20 or so blood, urine and other tests. When so many tests are done one or more abnormalities will be found in two thirds of all healthy individuals. Once an abnormal result has been obtained doctors feel obliged to continue doing tests. The tests they do often produce serious complications. Many patients who think they are ill – and have been told that they need to take drugs for life – are not really ill at all.
- Unnecessary tests are often done out of habit, for personal research, to provide protection in case of lawsuits or simply to impress other doctors. Doctors frequently order tests because it is quicker and easier to fill in a form than it is to talk to or examine a patient properly.
- When blood tests are done the results are compared against 'normal' values. But the 'normal' figures may have been produced decades earlier – by testing a few seemingly healthy doctors and nurses. No one really knows what is 'normal'. Your 'abnormal' result may be more 'normal' than the official 'normal' result.
- In Britain around 20,000 people a year get cancer from medical and dental X-rays.
- X-rays given to pregnant women during the 1950s and 1960s caused between 5% and 10% of all childhood cancers.
- Children who develop leukaemia – and other cancers – may have been made ill because their mothers had X-rays while they were pregnant.
- Doctors who know that tests can be misleading frequently order expensive, uncomfortable and even hazardous investigations – and then ignore the results.

I have dealt with the dangers of tests and investigations more fully in Chapter Nineteen of this book.

***

The interview is the most important part of the doctor's diagnostic equipment. That's when he talks to the patient and – even more important than talking though you wouldn't think so if you sit in on the average out-patients' clinic – listens to what the patient has to say. It is by talking to patients that doctors learn most.

Over the years doctors have accumulated more and more equipment to help them make diagnoses. But instead of helping, the equipment has come between the doctor and the patient. Too often the doctor relies exclusively on his damned equipment; trusting it implicitly to provide him with the right answers.

The first piece of equipment that doctors acquired was the stetho-scope. This now symbolic device was invented so that doctors could listen to their patients' chests without having to put their heads down on their bosoms. The stethoscope added to the doctor's dignity. But it also provided the first mechanical barrier between doctor and patient. And since René Laennec first introduced the stethoscope the doctor patient relationship has been weakened and damaged by this obsession with equipment and a failure to respect the relationship between doctor and patient.

A few years ago a study at Harvard University showed that one person in ten who had died would have still been alive if the doctors looking after them had relied upon their heads instead of their equipment.

One problem is the fact that the equipment doesn't allow for individual eccentricities.

Things are made even worse by the fact that equipment often breaks down and is frequently badly maintained. Shops have to have their scales calibrated but ask your doctor when he last had his blood pressure machine calibrated and watch him blush.

Checks showed that as much as half the new equipment being delivered to hospitals is defective. Indeed, can you think of any reason why the equipment that is supplied to hospitals should be any more reliable than the equipment you buy for your home?

If that doesn't worry you then the fact that many of the doctors who are responsible for using the equipment don't know how it works, how it should be calibrated or how to tell if it is working properly should worry you.

It is not uncommon for sales representatives to be present in operating theatres when equipment they have supplied is being used. They are there not just to give advice but to provide practical help. There are many people around who have been operated on not by surgeons but by sales representatives. I doubt if anyone knows how many patients the sales representatives have killed.

And who do you thinks trains doctors and nurses to operate all this wonderful, shiny new equipment? Often that is down to the sales representatives too.

***

Treatment is easy. You can look up treatment in five minutes. It's diagnosis that is difficult, and since the days of cupping and leeches it has been diagnostic skills which have differentiated between the good doctor and the bad doctor. Sadly, doctors have handed that particular art over to machinery – with disastrous results.

♦ When researchers examined the medical records of 100 dead patients who had been shown by post mortem to have had heart attacks they found that only 53% of the heart attacks had been diagnosed. What makes this even more alarming is the fact that half the patients had been looked after by cardiologists – experts in heart disease.

♦ A study of 32 hospitals which compared the diagnoses doctors had made when treating 1,800 patients with the diagnoses made after the patients had died (and could be examined more thoroughly) showed that doctors had an error rate of nearly 20%.

♦ A study of 131 randomly selected psychiatric patients showed that approximately three quarters of the patients may have been wrongly diagnosed.

♦ In many cases patients are diagnosed as having – and then treated for – serious psychiatric problems when their symptoms are caused by drugs they have been given for physical problems. Whole wards full of patients have been diagnosed, treated and classified as schizophrenic when in fact they were suffering from the drugs they had been given by prescription happy doctors.

♦ When 80 doctors were asked to examine silicone models of female breasts they only found half the hidden lumps. A 50% failure rate, even though the doctors knew that they were being tested and observed. The doctors spent an average of less than two minutes examining these false breasts for signs of cancer.

♦ Another study showed that doctors had missed diagnoses in dying patients up to a quarter of the time. Experts concluded that one in ten patients who had died would have lived if the correct diagnosis had been made.

♦ Another study revealed that in two thirds of patients who had died, important, previously undiagnosed conditions were first discovered in the post mortem room.

♦ A report published after pathologists had performed 400 post mortem examinations showed that in more than half the cases the wrong diagnosis had been made. The authors of this report said that potentially treatable disease was missed in 13% of patients; that 65 out of 134 cases of pneumonia had gone undetected and that out of 51 patients who had suffered heart attacks doctors had failed to diagnose the problem in 18 cases.

There are many reasons why today's doctors are so bad at making the correct diagnosis.

Education is often lamentable – with medical students taught about organs and tissues rather than living patients, and then examined on their ability to remember huge lists of details about bones, blood vessels and pathology details without being properly tested on their ability to use the information they have acquired.

Ignorance has become commonplace in medical practice.

A study of GPs reported in a medical newspaper a few years ago showed that a quarter of general practitioners did not know about the connection between smoking and heart disease while, amazingly, 20% of GPs were unaware that cigarettes could cause lung cancer. (One magazine editor refused to publish an article I wrote quoting this survey on the grounds that he couldn't believe that doctors could be so ignorant.) From France came evidence that in a final examination for medical students in Paris one tenth of the candidates made no mention of tobacco when asked to list factors responsible for causing cancer. By contrast, well over a third of the students mentioned the type of cancer produced in horses' mouths by the rubbing of the bit.

An even bigger problem is the fact that modern doctors rely far too much on technology – and far too little on building up any diagnostic skills of their own.

Old-fashioned doctors used to rely on what their patients told them and on what their own eyes, ears, noses and fingertips told them. Perhaps most important of all was the sixth sense that doctors acquired through years of clinical experience. Modern doctors rely too much upon equipment which is often faulty, frequently badly calibrated and more often than not downright misleading.

For example, nearly every published study on the subject puts the error rate for doctors reading X-rays at between 20% and 40%.

Radiologists working at a teaching hospital disagreed on the interpretation of chest radiographs as much as 56% of the time. And there were potentially significant errors in 41% of their reports.

Even when X-rays are read for a second time only about a third of the initial errors are spotted.

Two Irish doctors reported in the *British Medical Journal* that 20% of British patients who have slightly raised blood pressure are treated unnecessarily with drugs. Two pathologists who carried out several hundred post mortem examinations found that in more than 50% of the patients the wrong diagnosis had been made. An official report concluded that at least a fifth of all radiological examinations carried out in National Health Service hospitals were clinically unhelpful. In Britain it has been estimated that inexperienced doctors in casualty units kill at least one thousand patients a year.

***

Today, we have sophisticated diagnostic aids, monitoring systems, drugs, microscopic surgery, lasers and a thousand and one other miracles and yet we are, by and large, over cautious, hypochondriacal, drug abusing, overweight, neurotic, constipated, nervous, neurasthenic, hysterical and unhealthy. We are a tribute to and a product of our times.

When, to this appalling roll-call of largely doctor-induced disease you add the steadily increasing dissatisfaction with extended waiting lists, arrogant doctors, indifference and a lack of civility or caring it is hardly surprising that millions of people are today abandoning the traditional suppliers of medical help and seeking help from alternative practitioners.

***

Orthodox medical practitioners like to give the impression that they have conquered sickness with science but there are, at a conservative estimate, something in the region of 18,000 known diseases for which there are still no effective treatments – let alone cures. Even when treatments do exist their efficacy is often in question. A recent report concluded that 85% of medical and surgical treatments have never been properly tested.

As drug companies become increasingly aware that curing serious disease is beyond their capability (and, indeed, their desire – for why should drug companies, which make their money out of people being sick, want to make people well?), they spend more and more effort on finding drugs to improve life or performance in some vague way.

There can be little doubt that a former Director General of the World Health Organization got it absolutely right when he startled the medical establishment by stating that 'the major and most expensive part of medical knowledge as applied today appears to be more for the satisfaction of the health professions than for the benefit of the consumers of health care'. The evidence certainly supports that astonishing and apparently heretical view. Profits, not patients, are now the driving force which rule the medical profession's motives, ambitions and actions. Doctors don't seem to care any more. The passion has gone out of medicine.

***

In my view, the biggest single reason why the medical profession is killing so many people is its alliance with the pharmaceutical industry.

The myth that we live long and healthy lives thanks to the drug industry and the medical profession has increased our expectations. We no longer expect to fall ill. And we expect a magic solution when we do fall ill. We don't want to be bothered making any effort to stay healthy because we have been taught to have faith that if we fall ill then the medical men will be able to cure us.

Over 40% of the information doctors receive about the drugs they prescribe comes directly from drug company representatives and drug company leaflets. Well over 50% of the rest of the information they receive comes from medical journals and meetings which are sponsored by drug companies. In the mid-1970s, in my book *The Medicine Men*, I warned that the medical profession was being controlled by the drug industry and had no real right to call itself a profession. Today, there is no longer any doubt. Today, the drug industry owns the medical establishment and much of the medical profession.

It is widely accepted that the majority of illnesses do not need drug treatment. Most patients who visit a doctor neither want nor expect drug treatment. But at least eight out of ten patients who visit a general practitioner will be given a prescription (though growing numbers of patients do not take the drugs that are prescribed for them).

Sadly, the myth about our improving health is just that — a myth. We do not live longer or healthier lives than our predecessors. On the contrary although we consume greater and greater quantities of medicine than ever before more of us are ill today than at any time in history. On any day you care to choose, in just about any developed country you care to mention, over half the population will be taking a drug of some kind. A recent survey of 9,000 Britons concluded that one in three people are suffering from a long-standing illness or disability. Other surveys have shown that in any one fourteen day period 95% of the population consider themselves to be unwell for at least a few of those days. At no time in history has illness been so commonplace. We spend more than ever on health care but no one could argue that there is any less illness in our society.

***

Modern clinicians may use scientific techniques but in the way that they treat their patients they are still quacks and charlatans, loyal to existing and unproven ideas which are profitable, and resistant to new techniques and technologies which may be proven and effective.

The fact that a doctor may use a scientific instrument in his work does not make him a scientist — any more than a typist who uses a word processor is a computer scientist. The scientific technology available to doctors may be magnificent, but the problem is that the application of the scientific technology is crude, untested and unscientific.

Modern physicians and surgeons do not see the human mind and the human body as a single entity (which is why the medical profession has been slow to embrace the principles of holistic medicine and doubly incompetent in its attempts to deal with stress-related disorders) and they rely more on hopes and assumptions than on evidence and objective clinical experience. The modern clinician is as narrow-minded and as influenced by his personal experiences and interpretations as was his predecessor two thousand years ago.

Most patients probably assume that when a doctor proposes to use an established treatment to conquer a disease he will be using a treatment which has been tested, examined and proven. But this is not the case.

The *British Medical Journal* in October 1991 carried an editorial reporting that there are 'perhaps 30,000 biomedical journals in the world, and they have grown steadily by 7% a year since the 17th century.' The editorial also reported that: 'only about 15% of medical interventions are supported by solid scientific evidence' and 'only 1% of the articles in medical journals are scientifically sound'.

What sort of science is that? How can doctors possibly regard themselves as practising a science when six out of seven treatment regimes are unsupported by scientific evidence and when 99% of the articles upon which clinical decisions are based are scientifically unsound?

The savage truth is that most medical research is organised, paid for, commissioned or subsidised by the drug industry. This type of research is designed, quite simply, to find evidence showing a new product is of commercial value. The companies which commission such research are not terribly bothered about evidence; what they are looking for are conclusions which will enable them to sell their product. Drug company sponsored research is done more to get good reviews than to find out the truth.

A study published in the *Journal of the American Medical Association* found that one in five researchers in the life sciences had delayed publication of their results, or had not published them at all, because of their relations with business firms. Whenever I have accused scientists of being prejudiced and 'bought' because of their allegiance to their corporate paymasters the answer has invariably been the same: 'Everyone does it. There isn't a scientist in the world who hasn't taken corporate money.' This is probably true – and is one explanation for the fact that many allegedly independent government bodies are almost always packed with men and women who work for (or have taken fees from) the large corporations their government body is supposed to be policing.

It is also a fact that most of the doctors and scientists writing articles, papers and reviews for medical and scientific journals have received money, grants and freebies from drug, chemical or food companies. (It is also worth remembering that many allegedly and apparently independent journals accept corporate advertising and some accept payment in return for running articles.)

***

The absence of scientific evidence supporting medical practices is apparent in all areas of medicine.

With very few exceptions there are no certainties in medicine. The treatment a patient gets will depend more on chance and the doctor's personal prejudices than on science.

Even in these days of apparently high technology medicine there are almost endless variations in the treatments preferred by differing doctors.

Doctors offer different prescriptions for exactly the same symptoms; they keep patients in hospital for vastly different lengths of time, and they perform different operations on patients with apparently identical problems. The likelihood of a doctor accurately predicting the outcome of a disease is often no more than 50:50.

There is, indeed, ample evidence now available to show that the type of treatment a patient gets when he visits a doctor will depend not so much on the symptoms he describes but on the doctor he consults – and where that doctor practises.

Each year in America 61 in every 100,000 people have a coronary bypass operation. In Britain only about 6 in every 100,000 have the same operation. In Japan 1 in 100,000 patients will have a coronary bypass operation.

In America and Denmark seven out of every ten women will have a hysterectomy at some stage in their lives but in Britain only one woman in five will have the same operation. Why? Are women in America having too many hysterectomies or are women in Britain having too few?

In America 20% of babies are born by Caesarean delivery. In England and Wales the figure is 9%. In Japan 8% of confinements end in a Caesarean delivery.

Despite all these variations in the type of treatment offered most doctors in practice seem to be convinced that their treatment methods are beyond question. Many GPs and hospital doctors announce their decisions as though they are carved in stone.

***

The practice of medicine has become no more than an adjunct to the pharmaceutical industry and the other aspects of the huge, powerful and immensely profitable health care industry.

Medicine is no longer an independent profession.

✸ Doctors are no more dedicated to the saving of lives and the improvement of patients welfare than are the thousands of drug company salesmen and marketing men. Doctors have become nothing more than a link connecting the pharmaceutical industry to the consumer. ✸

It is not difficult to see why the drug industry behaves in such a ruthless manner. The profits to be made are phenomenal. It is not at all uncommon for a drug company to sell several hundred million dollar's worth of one product in a year. Companies can make 90 cents' pure profit for every dollar's worth of a drug that they sell. The raw materials for a drug may cost less than $100 a kilo. Turning the raw materials into 100,000 pills and packing them may take the total cost to $1,000. The retail price for 100,000 pills may be over $100,000. The only other internationally sold product that can compare for profitability is cocaine.

Drug companies frequently make minimum annual profits of between 30% and 50% on their capital employed. These profits, incidentally, come after massive marketing costs and payments to doctors.

Nor are profits likely to drop. The number of drugs doctors prescribe does not seem to be slowing down. A recent survey of over 2,000 patients admitted to hospital showed that within a ten year period the number of drugs prescribed per patient had shown an increase of almost 50%.

***

Occasionally politicians mutter about the obscene levels of drug company profits but the industry is efficient and ruthless and politicians are usually dealt with easily. The truth is that most politicians are, for a variety of reasons, reluctant to interfere with the drug industry. Drug companies which make money, provide jobs and pay taxes; in most developed countries they bring in revenue from abroad. Even the least effective drug company should be able to sell its products to developing countries.

✸ But the key factor in the failure of the politicians to control the drug industry is surely that neither politicians nor industrialists are particularly keen to see illness conquered. The drug industry wants to see as many people as possible suffering from long term, incurable illnesses. The politicians want to see people die before they become old and dependant. If more money was spent on preventing cancer (around 80% of cancers are preventable) then the average life expectancy would go up dramatically and the incidence of disease and disability would fall. But the drug industry doesn't want a healthy nation (it would sell fewer drugs) and the politicians don't want any more people living to an old age because they know that they would not be able to cope with the pensions bills they would have to pay. ✸

The medical establishment, which has sold its soul for pots of gold, and which is now controlled by an industry whose primary aim is to maximise the number of sick people in society, rarely criticises the drug industry. Most academic research departments, medical journals and medical associations rely heavily if not exclusively on the drug industry. The drug industry effectively owns the medical establishment.

***

I don't have faith in the medical establishment and I don't have much faith in the committees who give advice on health and food matters to our political leaders and to civil servants.

It is difficult to trust the conclusions and recommendations of official government committees or quangos because they are, inevitably, peopled by individuals who have been selected because they are compliant rather than complaining. Dissenters don't get picked to sit on committees to advise the government. In contrast the people who give out official guidelines on food and drugs are, more often than not, benefiting personally from the food and drug industries – and are, therefore, often benefiting financially from their own decisions.

Under those circumstances it isn't always easy to be certain that our politicians are acting on entirely impartial advice. The evidence of what these people have done in the last few decades could certainly not be used in their defence.

These days most government committees consist largely of individuals who work for or with the appropriate industries. An American newspaper, *USA Today*, recently expressed some surprise that 54% of 300 experts, sitting on 18 advisory committees, and hired to advise the US government on the safety and effectiveness of medicines, had a direct financial interest in the drug or subject they were being asked to evaluate.

Some of the experts received consulting fees, others had research grants from the companies they were supposed to be investigating and others had shares or stock options.

I found worse figures in the UK twenty or thirty years ago (though no British newspaper had the courage to print the findings).

Federal law prohibits the Food and Drug Administration in the US from using experts with financial conflicts but this law is often waived. (It has been waived more than 800 times since 1998.)

It is because our bureaucracies are controlled in this way that we have absurd regulations which are intended to protect the consumer but which, in reality, favour industry and do nothing for the consumers.

We have treaties which result in food surpluses being dumped. We have regulations which make the spread of Mad Cow Disease inevitable.

We have regulations which make it nigh on impossible for people to sell safe, effective remedies which might compete with drug company products. We have regulations requiring food companies to put additives and other chemicals into otherwise edible foods. We have genetic engineering hazards everywhere we look.

An American company has been given a patent in a type of rice. The peasants who perfected this variety of rice now cannot use it unless they pay the company holding the patent.

Global corporations, mostly American, now own many of the seeds of established crops. Peasants can no longer sow the seeds they save from the plants they grow. They must buy their seeds, every year, from big American seed companies. The peasants can't afford to do this. So the poor people in countries around the world starve to death unless they buy expensive food from American companies. Because they can't afford to pay those prices, governments and charities have to intervene and use your money and my money to help prevent mass starvation. Naturally, all this helps ensure the continued rising profits of these companies.

A generation ago the average dairy cow produced eight quarts of milk a day. Today, a typical cow produces fifty quarts a day. Just how do you think the farmers have changed nature so dramatically? Why haven't any government advisors asked questions?

A generation ago cows ate grass. Today cows may be fed blood and bone taken from other cows.

A generation ago milk was banned if it contained more than a trace of antibiotics. Today milk is stuffed with antibiotics and other drugs. One expert reports finding 52 different residues of antibiotics in a sample of milk in the US.

And who has allowed this to happen?

Those so-called independent experts who sit on committees and advise governments.

People who sit on committees allegedly regulating the products of the drug industry may not work full time for the drug industry but most of them have, or have had, lucrative contracts with drug companies. How absurd.

Whenever I have confronted politicians with the fact that members of powerful committees have drug company links they have responded by arguing that all doctors have drug company links and so it is impossible to find alternatives.

Free-thinking individuals who are not beholden to industry are never likely to find themselves sitting on any of these committees.

***

Antibiotics have been around for 40 years and the drug companies making them must have made billions of dollars in profits but no one yet knows how long antibiotic tablets should really be taken for when treating any specific condition. Should you take an antibiotic course for 5, 7, 10 or 14 days? The bizarre truth is that your guess is probably as good as your doctor's and his is probably as good as the drug company's.

Apart from failing to test its products properly there are several ways in which the drug industry shows that it is more concerned with profit than with healing the sick and conquering disease.

First, the vast majority of the 'new' drugs which the industry produces are not really offering anything new at all but are merely variations on existing themes.

According to the World Health Organization only about 200 drugs are essential. At any one time there will, however, be anything up to 30,000 drugs on the market (the precise figure varies from day to day and from country to country). Only 16% of the drugs sold by European pharmaceutical companies meet the World Health Organization definition of essential drugs. (The 16% comes to far more than 200 because, of course, there are numerous versions of each of the 'essential' drugs on the market.) Most of the non essential drugs will be duplicates produced by profit-hungry drug companies which want to share the world's most profitable markets. None of this will stop a drug company claiming that its new product is a life-saving miracle drug that must be allowed onto the market without delay.

Although it is firmly based in the developed world, the international drug industry will happily make whatever profits it can in the developing countries, marketing its products as unscrupulously as the tobacco giants.

Although drug companies spend virtually no money on studying the sort of diseases which afflict human beings in the developing countries they do, nevertheless, sell around 20% of the value of their combined drugs to the governments of those countries. The drug companies will admit that diseases which afflict the people of Africa and Asia aren't profitable enough to merit any research investment, but they will happily sell their expensive brand name versions of tranquillisers, sleeping tablets, pain killers, and the other pharmacological garbage of the developed world into those countries.

Moreover, when they sell into developing countries the drug companies, like the tobacco companies, can use advertising and marketing techniques which not even the lax governments of the West would allow.

Indeed, they don't just sell off products which are too dangerous for sale in the developed countries, they also use drugs in ways that would never be allowed in developed countries. For example, doctors in developing countries may be encouraged to prescribe drugs to help improve the growth of malnourished children who really just need better food.

There is a ruthlessness about the drug companies which makes the arms business look positively philanthropic. Drug companies have even been known to push up prices of drugs in small developing countries which have been hit by epidemics. To the drug industry, profit is everything.

Most doctors are obsessed with drug therapy. Many don't seem to have heard of the many effective non drug solutions which now exist. If it doesn't come in a blister pack and isn't packaged by one of the world's big drug companies they don't believe it can possibly work.

The big mistake most doctors make is to assume that drug companies are in business because they want to make sick people well again. That is a big, big mistake. The drug companies make drugs. That is what they do. But they make drugs so that they can make a profit. (And that they do very well – better, indeed, than probably any other industry.) Drug companies do not exist to help patients get better. They exist solely to make profits – they use sickness as a route to profit. And, to be frank, why should we expect them to be in business for any other reason?

Motor car companies aren't in business because they want to help people move around. They are in business because they think they can make a profit out of selling cars. Supermarkets aren't in business because they want to make shopping easier and cheaper. They are in business to make a profit. Arms companies don't make bombs and landmines because they want to help small, threatened countries defend themselves against aggressive neighbours. They make bombs and landmines because they can make big profits out of selling them.

I don't hate drug companies but I do think we need to regard them with great scepticism for they are (together with the food and tobacco industries) one of the three major modern threats to human health.

Doctors simply do not understand any of this. They wrongly assume that the drug companies have interests which match their own interests and which match the interests of their patients.

This is silly.

If doctors thought this through they would realise that patients and drug companies have diametrically opposed interests. The patient wants to get better. But the drug company will make bigger profits if the patient remains ill – and continues to need to take drugs.

But either through collective stupidity or through naivety (or because they like being bribed by drug companies) doctors like to believe that drug companies exist for the good of mankind.

Doctors should regard drug companies with scepticism and they should keep their relationship with them at arms length. They should regard drug companies as providing just one group of possible remedies.

But collectively doctors have behaved pretty stupidly. They have sold out to the drug industry and they have (as I pointed out more than 25 years ago in *The Medicine Men*) become little more than a marketing arm of the world's most profitable industry.

Drug companies have, not surprisingly, welcomed and taken advantage of the medical profession's collective stupidity (and/or naivety). They have virtually taken over postgraduate medical education. Their advertising dominates medical journals. And as a result most doctors (not just the bad ones) are obsessed with drugs because they simply aren't aware that there are other ways to deal with health problems.

I could give you dozens of examples of ways in which drug companies do things which are in their own financial interests but not in the interests of patients.

For example, in order to increase their profitability the drug companies are always looking for new ways to use existing products.

They do not do this because they want to help more people. They do it because they want to make bigger profits.

Consider, for example, the benzodiazepine tranquillisers.

Originally introduced specifically to help calm extremely nervous and agitated patients (and for use as anaesthetics) these drugs were, by the time they reached their peak, being prescribed for just about every illness known to man or woman. I met people who had been prescribed them as treatments for backache, menopausal problems, pre-menstrual tension, migraine, high blood pressure, alopecia and urinary tract infections.

It got to the point where doctors were handing out prescriptions for benzodiazepine tranquillisers whenever they didn't know what else to do. There was never any evidence to show that these drugs were effective in treating all these different conditions.

As a result it was hardly surprising that in the UK alone three million people became addicted to these drugs. (Benzodiazepine addiction was, and probably still is, the world's biggest drug addiction problem. Governments which spend billions on their wretched and pointless war against illegal drugs do it with the help of money which they raise from taxes on drug companies which are allowed to sell and promote drugs which are far more addictive than heroin, cocaine or cannabis.)

Similarly, look at what has happened with the drugs which were introduced for the treatment of arthritis.

Indomethacin and other powerful non-steroidal anti-inflammatory drugs (NSAIDs) worked well in the treatment of arthritis and helped relieve the pain, the stiffness and the swelling that occurs in conditions such as rheumatoid arthritis and gout where there is a lot of acute inflammation. Within a relatively short time there were dozens of competing products on the market.

But the drug companies wanted bigger profits than even the huge arthritis market would provide. And so they encouraged doctors to prescribe their products for headaches, period pains, and any other type of pain you can think of.

Doctors ignored the fact that these drugs didn't work terribly well for these conditions and they also ignored the fact that the side effects associated with these drugs were often more damaging than the conditions for which they were now being prescribed.

In both these examples (which are, incidentally, merely two of many) the failure of the drugs to work effectively, and the incidence of side effects, meant that patients lost faith. It was patients (not doctors) who expressed their unhappiness with these products.

The drug companies responded in the only sensible commercial way.

They introduced new drugs which did not have the side effects associated with the old, largely discredited drugs. Instead of recommending that doctors prescribe tranquillisers for millions of their patients they recommended that doctors prescribe anti-depressants. And instead of recommending non-steroidal anti-inflammatory drugs for every variety of pain the drug companies introduced new pain killers.

The drug companies spent a lot of money telling doctors that these drugs were new, effective and safe.

These drugs were new, but there wasn't any good evidence showing that they were effective or safe. Much of the evidence that existed was based on animal experiments and was irrelevant to human patients. Doctors didn't notice that. They wanted to look clever so they just started to prescribe the new drugs in vast quantities. Doctors are just as fashion conscious as any other consumer.

In due course the new drugs will invariably be found to have side effects of their own. After a few million people have taken the drugs for a few years the side effects will surface and will become more and more widely appreciated.

The drug companies (which will have made vast profits out of the drugs) will then, again, introduce something new.

Doctors should leave drug companies to get on with what they do best – making a profit. And they should do what they are trained and paid to do – look after patients.

Drugs can and often are useful and effective. They can be life-saving. But there are lots of ways to look after patients without using drugs.

And patients will only get good treatment when doctors realise that drug companies aren't on their side or on the side of patients. Drug companies are in the business of making money. That's what they do best.

***

Doctors have lost the breadth of vision to enable them to see opportunities for cure outside the traditional range of pharmacological opportunities.

The drug industry has convinced doctors that everyone they see must need a drug and that there is a pill for every ill. The majority of doctors might as well be employed directly by the drug companies, as pretend to be independent, authoritative scientists. They prescribe what they are told to prescribe in exactly the same way that the drug company representatives promote what they are told to promote.

The modern doctor would like to be regarded as a mystical healer; that, indeed, is how he probably sees himself in his dreams.

But in reality the modern doctor is little more than a drug company employee; pushing the latest line in wonder drugs with evangelical enthusiasm, never daring to criticise or to question the promotional material he is shown, grasping his free pen, golf ball or umbrella and wearily handing out the latest wonder drug until it is superseded by another wonder drug and imagining that by prescribing the latest new drug he is remaining on the frontiers of science and helping to push back the barriers of ignorance.

***

The fact that the medical profession is dominated and controlled by the pharmaceutical industry would not matter so much if the drug industry was honest, responsible and ethical. But it isn't. There is no other industry in the world which is as profitable or as ruthless as the drugs industry.

The pharmaceutical industry is (and has for many years been) the most consistently and astonishingly profitable industry in the world. The profits in this industry invariably put drug companies high up amongst the most financially successful companies in the world. The industry pays retainers and fat fees to a vast number of politicians, journalists and professional lobbyists and uses consequential power to keep its profits rising at a healthy rate. Even after all those fees and retainers the profits are massive.

In America since 1980 drug prices have risen at nearly six times the rate of other goods. When one drug is sold to treat animals the cost is $15 (possibly because animals aren't worth much and so the price can't be allowed to rise too high or else no one will buy the drug) but when the same drug is sold for the treatment of human patients the price rises to around $1,500.

For a long time now drug companies have enjoyed massive profits and their earnings have grown at the rate of 15%-20% a year. It is hardly surprising that the industry has for years been the brokers' favourite.

According to a survey published in the *Annals of Internal Medicine*, nearly two thirds of the pharmaceutical advertisements in medical journals are either grossly misleading or downright inaccurate. A total of 109 advertisements from 10 leading medical journals were each reviewed by two doctors and an academic clinical pharmacist. The reviewers used guidelines from the Food and Drug Administration to assess the advertisements. In 30% of cases the independent reviewers disagreed with the advertiser's claim that the drug was the drug of choice. In 44% of cases the reviewers thought that the advertisement would lead to improper prescribing if a doctor had no information about the drug other than that provided in the advertisement.

**

It can hardly be a surprise to anyone to realise that in some parts of the Western world – United States of America for example – more people now visit alternative practitioners for homoeopathy, acupuncture, osteopathy and so on, than visit traditional doctors. If you think about that it means that alternative medicine is no longer the alternative. Alternative medicine is the medical method of choice. Orthodox medicine is now the alternative. Alternative practitioners can now look down their noses at their orthodox colleagues in the same way that orthodox doctors have been looking down their noses for decades.

I firmly believe that the future clearly lies with an holistic approach which takes the best from all forms of medicine. It is crucial to remember that in a doctor-patient relationship only the interests of the patient are significant. I believe that the patient must take an active role in maintaining and restoring his or her own health and that the healing power of the mind and the body must be respected. I will explain the significance of holistic medicine more fully in the next chapter.

Chapter Four

Why You Should Learn To Be A Holistic Patient

Holistic (or, as it is sometimes spelt, wholistic) medicine has, for several decades, been growing in popularity. Many alternative and some orthodox health care professionals describe themselves as 'holistic' practitioners.

But they aren't.

Most journalists inaccurately assume that the word is a synonym for 'alternative' or 'complementary' medicine.

But it isn't.

The word 'holistic' was first introduced in 1926 by the South African philosopher and statesman Jan Christian Smuts. He suggested that the whole human being is much more than (and quite different to) a collection of physical or emotional parts. Even in those days, it seems, there must have been doctors parading up and down hospital wards referring to the 'liver' in the end bed and the 'case of pancreatitis' in the third bed on the left.

The word and the concept lay more or less forgotten until the 1970s when the growth of high technology medicine led to a revolution among patients who felt that aggressive, interventionist medicine wasn't entirely satisfactory. Suddenly there was a feeling that specialisation and fragmentation were not all they had been cracked up to be.

The use of the word 'holistic' meant, in theory at least, that instead of regarding patients as sick kidneys or hearts, health care professionals would try to meet the physical, mental, emotional and spiritual needs of their patients by dealing with social problems as well as physical ones, and by using natural healing methods as well as modern, pharmacological or surgical techniques.

In short, the word 'holistic' was intended to describe an attitude. An attitude which can just as well be followed by an orthodox trained doctor as by an alternative practitioner. A general practitioner in a busy city health centre can be holistic in his approach just as easily as can a herbalist or acupuncturist working from a back bedroom.

***

There is no doubt that a holistic approach to medical care is extremely good news for patients. When followed properly it means that every illness can be treated with a 'pick and mix' approach – choosing whichever aspects of orthodox and alternative medicine are most likely to be effective, and least likely to produce side effects, and taking full notice of all aspects of the individual's being.

In many illnesses there is no point in treating what is wrong with the body unless you also treat what is wrong with the mind . It seems to me remarkable that a modern doctor will treat the body of a patient who is suffering from high blood pressure, irritable bowel syndrome or asthma but ignore the mind, when it is now established beyond doubt that in so many illnesses the physical symptoms are produced by mental turmoil of one sort or another. It is equally bizarre and, in truth, unscientific, for an osteopath to treat a patient's back and ignore his mind.

The advantages of a truly holistic approach are colossal, not only because holistic medicine offers a chance to use the best and avoid the worst, but also because different types of treatment can, when used together, have a synergistic effect. A genuinely holistic approach may use a drug, a relaxation technique and massage to tackle a single collection of symptoms.

But although in theory the word 'holistic' implies an admirable change in attitude there is, sadly, little evidence that practitioners really understand what the word means or how it should be applied in practice.

It would be nice to think that everyone could find a holistic practitioner to look after them. But don't hold your breath. You've about as much chance of striking oil when digging in your winter vegetables.

***

Sadly, the steady rise in popularity of alternative medicine has made remarkably little impact on the way that orthodox medicine is practised. There are, it is true, a few orthodox practitioners who offer alternative forms of treatment (though, sadly, many of these are best described as dabblers rather than practitioners – there are people practising acupuncture, osteopathy, homoeopathy and hypnotherapy on the basis of one or two weekend courses) but the establishment view remains unchanged: alternative medicine is a dangerous waste of time and money which should be patronised when it cannot be ignored and suppressed whenever possible.

The myth that drug therapy offers the only true solution is now re-peated unquestioningly and without hesitation or embarrassment. Many members of the medical establishment believe that medical advance largely depends upon the pharmaceutical industry. This is not regarded as a subject for debate but as a fundamental building block; a fact of modern medical life.

The importance of drug therapy, and the reverence with which drugs are regarded by doctors and nurses, is perhaps best seen in modern rural health centres where doctors dispense as well as prescribe and where the dispensing counter where patients exchange their prescription slips for drugs is rather akin to a high altar. The modern consultation is, too often, a simple, thoughtless three-part process.

First, the patient visits the doctor and reports his or her symptoms. Second, the doctor decides which drug (or, more likely, which drugs) will be most appropriate and writes out what he considers to be an appropriate prescription. And third, the patient takes the prescription to the high priest and has it turned into a bottle of pills, a tube of ointment, an inhaler or whichever form has been deemed appropriate. An orthodox, modern medical school training means (literally) that a doctor is trained and kept up to date by and for the pharmaceutical industry. This may sound like hyperbole. It isn't. Drug companies pay for a very large part of the education that a doctor receives. Everyone in modern health care worships at the sterile shrine of the pharmacy.

It is not surprising, therefore, that the medical establishment still looks with horror at alternative medicine. Attempts to organise research programmes are invariably treated with a patronising dismissal.

It is one of the great modern scandals that the billion dollar worldwide 'charity' cancer industry, the international drug industry and the medical 'profession' (now, more of a trade than a 'profession') would all much rather suppress an alternative cancer treatment rather than have to admit that orthodox remedies might be bettered. The media supports this unholy trinity. In my book *Power over Cancer* (published by the European Medical Journal) I explained how 80% of cancer deaths could be avoided simply by avoiding factors (such as foods) which are known to cause cancer and eating foods which are known to provide protection from cancer. This, and my other attempts to educate the public about the real causes of cancer (and the best ways to tackle the disease), have been vilified or ignored by the cancer industry and the media (often working together).

The truth is that the medical establishment – and the drug industry – are terrified of alternative medicine for they regard it as a major commercial threat.

So, the bottom line is that you are unlikely to find a holistic orthodox practitioner after all.

***

You might expect to do better among alternative practitioners. But I fear that you would probably be disappointed there too. Tragically, too many alternative care practitioners are, in their complementary way, just as arrogant and intellectually isolated as medical men and women who have been trained to hand out pills.

Many acupuncturists, homoeopaths, herbalists and others describe themselves as offering their patients 'holistic' medicine when in reality they offer nothing of the sort.

However well trained she may be, the alternative therapist who confines herself to a single speciality is not a 'holistic' practitioner. How many acupuncturists, herbalists and naturopaths will admit that orthodox doctors and hospitals can sometimes provide the best care?

To be honest I don't think that many patients are ever going to receive truly 'holistic' treatment from their practitioners – whether they are orthodox or alternative. Most training programmes are, by their very nature, designed to produce specialists. Medical schools turn out drug dispensers and acupuncture schools turn out acupuncturists. And there aren't many health care professionals with the time or inclination to study other available specialities.

We must also recognise that there is, of course, a huge financial disincentive involved here. How many practitioners are going to suggest to a paying patient that he would obtain better treatment by visiting another professional? I know of very few truly 'holistic' centres where a patient can obtain treatment from a comprehensive variety of orthodox and alternative practitioners.

All this is sad.

But it doesn't mean that holistic medicine is out of reach.

What it does mean is that if you really want holistic treatment (and in my opinion you should) you're going to have to take control yourself if you or anyone in your family needs treatment.

There are very few truly holistic medical practitioners. But everyone can – and should – be a holistic patient. Anyone who is ill needs attention to their mind and spirit as well as their body. Selecting a properly balanced diet may be as important as choosing the right drug. Sometimes a successful outcome to an illness may be 80% dependent on choosing the right drug. On another occasion a successful outcome may be 80% dependent on diet.

Holistic practitioners are rare – but you can and should be a holistic patient.

Chapter Five

Orthodox or Alternative: Which is Best?

When is orthodox treatment best? What can doctors offer if you want to avoid getting heart disease? Are the alternative remedies for irritable bowel syndrome better − or worse − than orthodox treatments? If you're suffering from anxiety is your doctor likely to offer more effective help than an alternative practitioner?

These − and questions like them − are questions which really matter, and which have a real influence on your chances of longevity.

I have, therefore, taken a hard, critical look at the ways in which orthodox and alternative practitioners claim to be able to prevent − and treat − ten of the commonest diseases. This chapter is an independent and personal assessment and evaluation of the comparative effectiveness of alternative and orthodox medicine in the treatment of ten common diseases.

I readily admit that this comparison of orthodox and alternative medicine is inevitably subjective to a certain extent. But I have based my conclusions on the available evidence and since I am not influenced by any outside forces (politicians, corporate interests or loyalty to any particular section of the healing community) I have made the study as objective as I possibly could.

I have given both orthodox medicine and alternative medicine a general score at the end of each section.

I do realise that individual practitioners will score very differently within these two categories; my scoring is intended to recognise the general value of the help available from practitioners.

I also added a score for 'self-help' since it is often possible for the

71

informed individual to keep him/herself healthy (and to restore good health) far more effectively without professional help than with it.

Anxiety and depression

Prevention

Your doctor is unlikely to offer you any help in avoiding anxiety or depression. This is one of many areas of orthodox medicine where 'prevention' is a concept which really does not exist. Alternative practitioners are a little better. Some practitioners may offer stress counselling and relaxation therapy (both of which would undoubtedly help improve mental health and reduce the likelihood of both anxiety and depression) and others will offer nutritional advice which may be of value since there is no doubt that a poor diet can (largely through leading to a poor immune system) lead to an increased susceptibility to stress.

Score

Orthodox medicine	0/10
Alternative medicine	4/10
Self-help	7/10

Treatment

The commonest orthodox treatment for both anxiety and depression involves drug therapy. Tranquillisers are the usual choice for anxiety despite the fact that they offer only superficial, temporary support and can produce serious problems of their own.

After the problems associated with tranquilliser use were acknowledged the pharmaceutical industry and the medical profession (predictably) concentrated their efforts on marketing anti-depressants. Anti-depressants do seem to help some patients but, once again, there are numerous side effects – some of them serious.

Psychotherapy is the second most popular treatment for anxiety or depression but because of the high cost it is not available to most patients. This may not be too much of a disadvantage since there is some evidence to suggest that support provided by friends and acquaintances may be more useful than professional support offered by psychiatrists, psychologists or therapists.

Surprisingly, perhaps, some doctors still recommend brain surgery for problems of this type. Patients who undergo destructive brain surgery may well behave differently (and may, therefore, be thought to have been 'cured' of their anxiety or depression) but my personal view is that this type of treatment is unacceptable. Chopping patients heads off would undoubtedly stop them feeling anxious or depressed but this is not a remedy I would recommend.

Alternative therapies for depression are mostly gentle, and seem relatively free of side effects, and they do seem to me to be probably safer than orthodox remedies. The effectiveness of the herb St John's Wort in the treatment of depression has been disputed but is popular and other forms of alternative medicine which may prove effective include nutritional therapies (including vitamin supplements), relaxation exercises, homoeopathy and Tai Chi.

Naturopathy (usually recommending a low intake of caffeine and alcohol and a decent intake of complex carbohydrates to stabilise blood sugar levels), hypnotherapy, relaxation exercises, meditation, massage and homoeopathy are forms of alternative medicine which may be useful in the treatment of anxiety.

Score

Orthodox medicine	3/10
Alternative practitioners	8/10
Self-help	8/10

Arthritis

Prevention

There is no orthodox prevention programme for arthritis. In the alternative medicine field the best prevention programme is the one offered by nutritionists who recommend a vegetarian diet. It has been proved that rheumatoid arthritis is less common among vegetarians than among meat eaters but, sadly, very few doctors providing advice to their patients on the subject of arthritis consider this link worth mentioning. (This may be because they are not aware of it. This ignorance is best explained by the fact that most doctors obtain their postgraduate education courtesy of the pharmaceutical industry which is, not surprisingly perhaps, interested exclusively in promoting the idea that drug therapy is the only sensible way of dealing with health problems and in advocating specific therapies within that genre.)

Score

Orthodox medicine	0/10
Alternative practitioners	6/10
Self-help	6/10

Treatment

The commonest orthodox treatment for arthritis involves drug therapy –

usually with non-steroidal anti-inflammatory drugs. The best established (and possibly the most effective) drug for the treatment of arthritis is aspirin, but this drug is not widely used by doctors partly because it is out of patent (and therefore made very cheaply by a large number of companies) and partly because it has acquired a bad reputation for causing stomach problems. Ironically, however, new (and invariably much more expensive) variations on this pharmacological theme usually turn out to cause similar symptoms when they have been on the market for a few years. The drug industry gets round this problem by producing a constant stream of new products. It is worth noting that soluble aspirin is much less likely to cause stomach problems than the non-soluble variety.

Drug therapy can help relieve some of the pain and stiffness associated with arthritis but that's about it. Astonishingly, most doctors are still unaware of just how effective TENS machines can be in eradicating the sort of pain suffered by patients with arthritis. Actually, it probably isn't all that astonishing since drug companies have, over the years, worked pretty hard to make sure that doctors continue prescribing drugs (very profitable for drug companies) and don't recommend TENS machines (no profit at all for drug companies). Back in the 1980s, when I first started writing about TENS machines, I reported that one drug company had bought a company making small but effective TENS machines. For about thirty seconds or so I thought that this was good news and that the drug company would now start promoting TENS machines. But the TENS machine company closed down. Surgery is the second most popular orthodox treatment for arthritis. The replacement of arthritic joints has become big business and seems destined to become an even bigger money-spinner in the future.

There are numerous 'alternative' remedies for arthritis but (unless you count the TENS machine as an 'alternative' remedy) the best of them are probably no better than the remedies offered by orthodox practitioners. Acupuncture may help relieve the pain of arthritis but it won't cure it any more than drugs will. Other useful alternative treatments for arthritis include nutritional ones (such as those advocated by naturopaths). Cutting out meat and fat and increasing the intake of fruit, vegetables and wholegrain cereals is likely to help. Hydrotherapy (regulated exercise in water) can help when joints are swollen or painful and homoeopathy may also prove useful.

Score

Orthodox medicine	5/10
Alternative practitioners	6/10
Self-help	7/10

Asthma

Prevention

Doctors claim that there has been an explosion in the incidence of asthma in recent years. You might, therefore, imagine that the medical profession would be looking for ways to prevent asthma. You would be disappointed. It is usually claimed that asthma is becoming commoner because of the pollutants in the air we breathe. I'm not entirely convinced by this argument. After all, our air has been polluted for a long time. I rather suspect that what is happening is that asthma is simply being diagnosed more enthusiastically because doctors are being pushed to prescribe anti-asthma drugs. If a child visits a doctor with a wheeze the doctor will diagnose asthma and start a treatment programme which may well last for life. This is patently absurd but none the less enormously profitable.

Some doctors do perform skin tests in a search for allergens which might be responsible. But most don't bother.

The best way to prevent asthma is, I believe, to teach people how to relax. Much asthma is stress related and learning how to relax when under pressure is an excellent way to abort a potential asthma attack. Sadly, the orthodox medical profession hardly ever bothers to do this. Some alternative practitioners do.

It is also important to remember that asthma can be caused by house dust mites, dander (tiny pieces of animal hair, skin and feathers), tobacco smoke, exhaust fumes and mould. Some food additives can also cause asthma. Good practitioners advise that the best way to avoid these varieties of allergic asthma is to avoid the allergens. Regretfully, alternative practitioners of various kinds are more likely to make this type of recommendation than are orthodox practitioners.

Score

Orthodox medicine	1/10
Alternative practitioners	6/10
Self-help	6/10

Treatment

Inhalers which contain drugs which dilate the air passages (broncho-dilators) are the cornerstone of orthodox treatment for asthma. Steroids are also popular – despite the possible side effects. There is no doubt that inhalers can be extremely effective – and as a result many users become very dependent upon them (the dependence is psychological rather than physical but none the less the real for that). But are inhalers always necessary? I don't think so. Many patients overuse them and are encouraged to overuse them by over-prescribing. Indeed, my fear is that the damage done by these drugs may outweigh the useful effects.

There is, in comparison, good evidence showing that asthma sufferers who are taught how to relax can deal very effectively with their symptoms, without any risk of side effects.

I have seen children and adults suffering from quite serious asthma make remarkable recoveries when helped to relax and I have no doubt that if more patients were taught to relax the need for inhalers would drop dramatically. (But so would drug company profits of course.)

Score

Orthodox medicine	5/10
Alternative practitioners	6/10
Self-help	6/10

Cancer

Prevention

The original and traditional orthodox medicine approach to preventing cancer was to create a new speciality which, perhaps not surprisingly, involved patients handing over fairly vast amounts of money to be 'screened' at regular but artificially defined intervals. The evidence suggests that this type of preventive medicine programme probably did more harm than good – except to the bank balances of the doctors and health companies organising it. One problem is that selective screening not infrequently produces false positives – which results in patients receiving therapy they don't need. Another problem is that screening programmes may create health problems of their own. (For example, X-ray screening may increase the risk of cancer developing and there has to be a serious risk that mammography, for example, may increase the risk of women developing breast cancer.) A third problem is that individuals who are screened annually may be imbued with a false sense of confidence – and may, therefore, ignore warning signs which they would have otherwise noticed.

Recently, the drug industry and the medical profession have combined to create a new and even more profitable form of 'preventive' medicine which involves the prescribing of powerful drugs which are intended to prevent cancer developing. Doctors and their drug company paymasters have realised that if they can persuade millions of patients to take drugs regularly in order to reduce their chances of developing a specific illness the profits will be spectacular – even by drug company standards.

The best known drug in this new category is tamoxifen. Women are being encouraged to take the drug to reduce their chances of developing cancer. When I first found out about this new development five or six years ago I warned that tamoxifen is known to cause uterine cancer. This revelation was acknowledged but dismissed by doctors and drug companies. Other side effects associated with tamoxifen are so significant that it is not uncommon for doctors to prescribe additional drugs to help alleviate them. Few orthodox doctors, or drug company representatives, seem to think it odd to give a perfectly healthy woman a cancer-causing drug to prevent cancer – and to then give another potentially harmful drug to alleviate other side effects.

Some surgeons have also moved into the world of 'preventive medicine'. It is becoming common for surgeons to remove healthy breasts from healthy women on the grounds that if there is no breast there then breast cancer is unlikely to develop.

Finally, of course, some doctors do make some effort to persuade patients who smoke to give up or reduce their consumption of tobacco (known to be a carcinogenic substance).

The alternative approach to preventing cancer is, it seems to me, considerably more logical than the so-called 'orthodox' approach which I have described.

We now know what causes 80% of all cancers and the main thrust of the approach advocated by the best alternative practitioners is to suggest to people who wish to cut their risk of developing cancer that they avoid as many carcinogens as possible – and that they should adapt their lifestyle in such a way as to minimise their chances of developing cancer. (Written down this sounds absurdly simple and it is difficult to believe that most members of the medical establishment would classify this approach as controversial.)

Apart from tobacco (virtually the only recognised carcinogen to be accepted by the medical establishment) the other known cancer inducing substances include a number of widely consumed foods. It is, for example, now proven beyond any shadow of doubt that meat causes cancer. There is also evidence showing that a high fat diet increases the risk of cancer developing. Removing meat and excess fat from the diet should, therefore, reduce the cancer risk. It is also known that eating more fruit and vegetables provides a good deal of protection against cancer and there is evidence to show that individuals who are overweight are more likely to develop cancer.

This lifestyle approach (based on existing clinical evidence) is so logical that it seems rather bizarre to have to acknowledge that it is still regarded as 'alternative' and, indeed, rather revolutionary. Good alternative practitioners will advise their healthy patients to avoid the foods which are known to cause cancer.

Cancer rates continued to rise throughout the twentieth century (and seem certain to continue to rise in the twenty first century). It would be hard to find more convincing evidence proving that the orthodox approach to preventing cancer has failed dismally.

Score

Orthodox medicine	0/10
Alternative medicine	8/10
Self-help	9/10

Treatment

The orthodox approach to the treatment of cancer consists of three separate types of therapy: chemotherapy, radiotherapy and surgery. The effectiveness (or otherwise) of this approach is easily measured by studying survival rates. And, as with preventive medicine, the evidence shows that the medical establishment has been appallingly unsuccessful.

Chemotherapy is one of the great health scandals of our time. Although hugely profitable for the pharmaceutical industry the evidence strongly suggests that, for the majority of cancers and the majority of patients, chemotherapy simply does not work. Indeed, I am convinced that because of the damaging effect it has on the immune system chemotherapy probably does more harm than good for many patients. There are occasions when chemotherapy is of value but I have no doubt whatsoever that if chemotherapy was an 'alternative' remedy it would have been banned as unsafe and ineffective. Doctors persevere with chemotherapy because they are taught (by the drug industry) that it is the most effective way to tackle cancer. Radiotherapy and surgery are equally controversial and although there are times when both can be of use the fact is that if they were 'alternative' remedies they too would have almost certainly been banned on the twin grounds of danger and ineffectiveness.

There are numerous alternative remedies for cancer available. But the basic principle of all the successful therapies I've found has been a low fat, vegetarian diet which includes plenty of vegetables and plenty of fruit – preferably consumed as juices. The evidence I have seen has convinced me that this dietary approach – either alone or with other therapies – is the most effective way to defeat cancer. And there is a logical explanation for this therapy since the high vitamin content of fruit and vegetables undoubtedly boosts the body's immune system.

The dietary approach to the treatment of cancer isn't the only type of therapy that works. Visualisation is undoubtedly also effective and is one of the most effective alternative solutions. As I showed in my books *Bodypower* and *Mindpower* back in the 1980s (now both published by the European Medical Journal) it is possible to defeat cancer by imagining that your body is full of cancer eating cells.

Score

Orthodox medicine	1/10
Alternative medicine	8/10
Self-help	8/10

Eczema and Dermatitis ✦

Prevention

A few orthodox practitioners may encourage susceptible patients to avoid irritants likely to cause eczema or dermatitis. But the vast majority do not – even though it isn't difficult to compile a shortlist of the most likely causes (nickel, rubber, sticking plaster, chemicals and household plants can cause allergic contact eczema; eggs and dairy produce can cause allergic eczema; oils can cause occupational eczema; soaps, detergents and urine can cause irritant eczema). There will be exceptions but I doubt if the majority of alternative practitioners are much better in this area than the majority of orthodox practitioners. However, individuals who avoid allergens and irritants will be able to protect themselves quite effectively.

As a footnote it is worth drawing attention to the fact that some cases of eczema may be produced by drugs (such as penicillin and sulphonamide) which have been taken by mouth. Doctors could, therefore, prevent a good deal of eczema by limiting their over-prescribing.

Score

Orthodox medicine	0/10
Alternative medicine	0/10
Self-help	6/10

Treatment

The orthodox treatment for eczema and dermatitis usually involves a steroid cream. Such creams will often prove effective – in the short term – but they do not, of course, deal with the underlying cause of the problem.

Orthodox practitioners can probably produce a miracle result more speedily than alternative practitioners but good alternative practitioners who spend a little time trying to find a cause for an attack of eczema will be much more likely to find a permanent solution. In practice most people will be able to solve this problem just as quickly as any alternative practitioner.

It is, incidentally, worth remembering that the sort of creams usually favoured by orthodox practitioners can actually cause eczema if used for too long.

Score

Orthodox medicine	5/10
Alternative medicine	8/10
Self-help	8/10

Headaches and Migraines

Prevention

Headaches are among the commonest of all health problems. And yet I doubt if most doctors ever give a thought to their prevention. The vast majority of headaches are 'tension headaches' – caused by stress and anxiety – and the best way to prevent headaches of this type is to learn how to deal with stressful situations more effectively. Learn how to spot when you are under too much pressure, and know how to wind down or shut yourself away from the pressures of a difficult world, and you should suffer far less from stress-related tension headaches. Learning how to relax your mind (and your body) isn't particularly difficult. It is a skill which (like dancing, driving a car or playing golf) needs to be learned. What a pity it is that doctors seem to be too busy to teach their patients how to do these things. Fortunately, there are some alternative practitioners around who are enthusiastic about teaching their patients these skills. Most important of all these are skills which can be learned at home without a practitioner of any kind. (*cf* my book *How To Relax and Overcome Stress*, published by the European Medical Journal.)

Migraine headaches are often linked to specific foods, or to other lifestyle factors, and they can, therefore, be prevented more easily than other types of headaches. Doctors will (occasionally) provide their patients with a list of possible triggers (cheese, chocolate and tobacco smoke are examples of known triggers).

Score

Orthodox medicine	1/10
Alternative medicine	6/10
Self-help	7/10

Treatment

Visit a doctor complaining of a headache and he will almost certainly reach for his prescription pad, scribble for a moment and send you off to the local pharmacy to pick up a bottle of painkillers. There is no doubt that painkillers will probably help. But they won't do anything to deal with the cause of the headache. They won't help you to deal with the problem yourself. And they won't help you avoid the problem occurring again. Giving a patient a painkiller to deal with a headache is like giving a motorist a bucket of water when his radiator is leaking. It's a short-term solution. When headaches persist, recur or are in some other way clearly out of the ordinary, doctors can do a good job in helping to make a diagnosis. But in the treatment of routine headaches orthodox doctors are pretty useless.

Massage, acupressure, homoeopathy and relaxation therapy are just a few of the alternative methods which may work in the treatment of headaches.

But the nature of the disorder means that self-help offers by far the best approach. Self-help treatment for headaches doesn't simply involve taking the top off the bottle of soluble aspirin and popping two tablets into a glass of water. Learning to relax, mastering the simple art of fingertip massage and controlling your exposure to stress are all crucial. Visualisation is a simple but effective way to deal with migraine. (I describe a powerful and effective technique in my book *Bodypower* published by the European Medical Journal.)

Score

Orthodox medicine	3/10
Alternative medicine	6/10
Self-help	9/10

Heart disease

Prevention
Doctors do make some effort to prevent heart disease but readers may not be too surprised to hear that most doctors regard drugs as the best way of doing this. Whether these drugs are effective is another question. And I certainly don't think that drugs of any kind are the best way to prevent heart disease.

Numerous studies have identified the causes of heart disease. They include: too much stress, being overweight, drinking too much alcohol, cigarette smoking, eating a fat rich diet, taking too little exercise and so on. Simple lifestyle changes can dramatically alter an individual's chances of developing heart disease. Alternative practitioners who can perform effectively in this area usually do so by recommending these lifestyle changes.

Score

Orthodox medicine	2/10
Alternative medicine	6/10
Self-help	9/10

Treatment

The orthodox treatment of heart disease usually involves either drugs or surgery – or a mixture of both. And yet there is clear evidence to show that drugs and surgery are not the best way to deal with this heart disease.

If doctors were true scientists and were genuinely devoted to offering their patients the best remedy for their problem then they would offer patients the type of solution tested and proven by Dr Dean Ornish and his colleagues.

Dr Ornish has shown that patients with heart disease can be cured by a programme consisting of a mixture of exercise, a low fat vegetarian diet, stress reduction and counselling. The research he has published (*Dr Dean Ornish's Program for Preventing Heart Disease* published by Ballantine Books, New York), is totally convincing. Some aspects of this programme can be followed at home by any intelligent reader although I have to warn patients that they must not stop medical treatment without first discussing things with their doctor, that I do not recommend that anyone begin any treatment for a heart condition without first obtaining advice from a qualified medical practitioner and that it is vital that anyone planning to follow this type of approach should first check with their doctor that the approach is appropriate for them.

Medically-approved and supervised self-help can be tremendously effective. Any doctor who insists that the only way to treat heart disease is with drugs or surgery is incompetent and should be promoted to cleaning the public lavatories. Although Dr Ornish and his colleagues are orthodox practitioners I don't feel I can include their treatment regime in my assessment of orthodox medicine since most doctors still prefer to recommend drugs or surgery. Alternative solutions for heart trouble include those offered by naturopathy, relaxation therapies, meditation and Tai Chi.

Score

Orthodox medicine	2/10
Alternative medicine	5/10
Self-help	8/10

High Blood Pressure

Prevention

High blood pressure is one of the easiest diseases to prevent. Too much stress, too much weight, too much fat in the diet – all these are among the avoidable factors.

Some doctors make an effort with some of their patients. But most orthodox doctors don't even bother to take routine blood pressure measurements – let alone give their healthy patients advice on how to avoid high blood pressure. Some alternative practitioners (particularly those with an interest in relaxation therapies and good nutrition) may teach patients how to avoid this problem. (For more information see my book *High Blood Pressure* published by the European Medical Journal.)

Score

Orthodox medicine	0/10
Alternative practitioners	4/10
Self-help	9/10

Treatment

The orthodox approach to the treatment of high blood pressure usually involves drug therapy. High blood pressure is one of the diseases drug companies love. Once a patient has high blood pressure he will (unless he makes changes to his lifestyle) often have it for life. That means that he will need pills for life. Drug companies love disorders like this. Drugs used in the treatment of high blood pressure frequently do bring the blood pressure down but they may cause unpleasant side effects. Tai Chi, meditation, visualisation and naturopathy are all varieties of alternative medicine which can prove effective. But the best way to tackle this problem is often to make lifestyle changes. (Patients – particularly those already receiving orthodox therapy – must talk to their doctor before making any lifestyle changes because the effectiveness of lifestyle changes can be so dramatic that medication may need to be altered.)

Score

Orthodox medicine	3/10
Alternative practitioners	5/10
Self-help	8/10

Irritable Bowel Syndrome

Prevention

Neither doctors nor alternative medicine practitioners do much to help individuals avoid irritable bowel syndrome (IBS). The sad truth is that many alternative practitioners aren't much better than orthodox doctors at telling patients how to stay healthy. The reason for this is obvious: both alternative practitioners and orthodox doctors get paid for treating sick patients, and they usually get paid for prescribing a specific remedy – whether it is a drug, a massage, a needle or a herb. Alternative medicine and orthodox medicine are both variations on the same interventionist theme. Having said this some alternative practitioners do recognise that IBS is usually caused either by stress or by dietary problems.

Score

Orthodox medicine	1/10
Alternative practitioners	3/10
Self-help	8/10

Treatment

Orthodox doctors, and most alternative practitioners, fail to offer IBS sufferers particularly good advice. Most are too keen to sell a product of some kind – even though the answer to IBS may be rather simpler than this practice might suggest. The fact is that IBS is usually caused by either stress or a diet problem.

It isn't possible to cure irritable bowel syndrome but it is usually possible to control it by teaching the patient how to deal with these two different problems. (Stress is best countered by reducing the exposure to unnecessary stresses while at the same time learning to relax and improving the ability to deal with stress. Dealing with the dietary link usually involves such simple remedies as cutting out dairy produce, reducing fat intake and increasing the intake of water.)

Orthodox doctors prescribe a wide range of pills for IBS sufferers. If a patient suffers from diarrhoea then a doctor will prescribe a pill to treat the diarrhoea. If the patient suffers from constipation then a laxative will be prescribed. Anti-spasmodics are popularly prescribed, as are medicines containing peppermint or charcoal (products which are also popular with alternative practitioners).

Many alternative practitioners are really no better than orthodox doctors when it comes to the treatment of irritable bowel syndrome. Many have a remedy to offer but relatively few offer 'lifestyle' advice which will really make a difference. Prescribing peppermint, fennel tea or charcoal may well help deal with the symptoms (and that can be very welcome), but won't reduce the incidence or extent of irritable bowel syndrome. (See my book *Relief from IBS* published by the European Medical Journal for more advice.)

Score:

Orthodox medicine:	2/10
Alternative medicine:	2/10
Self-help	8/10

Osteoporosis

Prevention

Most orthodox medical practitioners don't seem to understand how osteoporosis develops. They do very little to prevent it. Nor am I particularly impressed by the ability of alternative practitioners to help prevent osteoporosis. Individuals can, however, do a great deal to protect themselves from this problem. There are notes on building strong bones and avoiding osteoporosis in my book *Food For Thought* published by the European Medical Journal.

Score

Orthodox medicine	0/10
Alternative medicine	0/10
Self-help	9/10

Treatment

Generally speaking, orthodox medical practitioners are as terrible at treating osteoporosis as they are at preventing it. Many believe the myths about osteoporosis which have been sustained by those with corporate interests to promote. Most alternative medical practitioners aren't much better than orthodox practitioners at treating osteoporosis. The self-help solution is, in my view, the best answer.

Osteoporosis is a nasty disease but it is largely created and sustained by our way of life. As with so many other disorders our modern 'in a bottle' solutions often simply add additional problems to existing ones. The best way to avoid osteoporosis, and to deal with it, is to be aware of the real causes and to do something about them. Osteoporosis is yet another lifestyle disease which can best be avoided and conquered through a change in lifestyle.

Score

Orthodox medicine	0/10
Alternative medicine	0/10
Self-help	9/10

Conclusion

My general conclusion is that orthodox medicine has lost its way. The advice offered by doctors is too often self serving and too many practitioners offer only what they have been taught to offer (usually by drug companies). Drug companies aren't interested in teaching doctors how to use non-drug remedies and they aren't interested in defeating disease.

Why should they be?

Drug company profits depend upon large numbers of the population remaining permanently sick.

Alternative practitioners aren't immune to criticism either. Many who call themselves 'holistic practitioners' are no more 'holistic' than surgeons or radiotherapists. The herbalist who claims to be able to treat every ailment that comes his way with herbs is not a holistic practitioner. The acupuncturist who sticks rigidly to his needles is as narrow minded as any prescription-scribbling general practitioner. The branch of alternative medicine which seems to me to be closest to a truly holistic approach is naturopathy. Naturopaths emphasise a number of nutritional approaches which have been proven to be effective (and they sometimes recommend chocolate as a mood enhancer which is pretty darned sensible of them).

A careful analysis of the prevention and treatment programmes available suggests to me that the vast majority of the health problems in the developed world could be prevented, or treated, with a change in lifestyle. A healthy immune system is the key to good health, and yet most people do everything they possibly can to batter and weaken their immune systems. And neither doctors nor alternative practitioners do much to counteract this dangerous trend. The tragedy is that most doctors are keen to push pills, most acupuncturists are keen to push acupuncture, most herbalists are keen to push herbal remedies and so on. Truly holistic medicine is a rarity and encouraging people to make lifestyle changes isn't a very profitable occupation.

Chapter Six

How You Can Get The Best Out Of Your Doctor

Doctors are now a major cause of illness and death. Study the statistics and it becomes clear that throughout the 'civilised' world doctors are right up there alongside heart disease and cancer as the big-time killers of our time.
Here are ten reasons why you shouldn't trust your doctor:

1. He will have almost certainly been educated by drug companies anxious to sell their products – regardless of the side effects.
2. He may not know who you are – and may confuse you with someone else.
3. He may be using you as a guinea pig in a clinical trial. If your doctor gives you a packet of tablets (instead of a prescription) then the chances are high that he's being paid to test out a new drug.
4. He may well be sadly out of date. Most doctors are out of date within five years of leaving medical school.
5. He may be an alcoholic or a drug addict. Few groups of people turn to alcohol or drugs more often than doctors.
6. He probably has no idea what side effects may be associated with the drug he/she is prescribing.
7. He will almost certainly want to prescribe a drug for your symptoms – regardless of the fact that other methods of treatment may be both safer and more effective.
8. He may be relying on test results which are wrong – or which he simply doesn't understand. Errors involving tests and investigations are much commoner than most patients (and most doctors) realise. Most tests aren't as reliable, as useful or as necessary as most people think.

9. He may be depressed and in no fit condition to make a diagnosis or prescribe treatment. Mental illness is commoner among doctors than almost any other group in our society.
10. He may make treatment decisions based on his/her own religious beliefs – even though those personal beliefs mean that you do not receive the most appropriate treatment. The doctor is unlikely to tell you that his/her decisions are being affected in this way.

***

A study in Australia showed that 470,000 Australian men, women and children are admitted to hospital every year because they have been made ill by doctors. The figures also show that every year 280,000 patients who are admitted to hospital suffer a temporary disability as a result of their health care. Around 50,000 of these suffer permanent disabilities. A staggering 18,000 Australians die annually as a result of medical errors, drug toxicity, surgical errors and general medical mismanagement. What a terrible indictment of the medical profession.

In America the death rate from medical 'accidents' is running at around 200,000 a year. Figures in Europe are no better. In my book *Betrayal of Trust* I reported that one in six British hospital patients are in hospital because they have been made ill by doctors.

I could go on and on with figures and back it all up with plenty of evidence. The story is the same the whole world over and doctors no longer seem to deny any of this. When I was last invited onto a radio programme to talk about the fact that one in six patients in hospital are there because doctors have made them ill a doctor representing the medical establishment came into the studio to defend his profession. He argued that patients could take comfort from the fact that the figures showed that five out of six hospital patients were *not* sick because they had been made ill by doctors. (No, I could hardly believe it either. But I listened to a tape of the programme afterward and that is exactly what he said.)

Around half of all the 'adverse effects' associated with doctors are readily preventable and are usually a result of ignorance or incompetence or a mixture of both. The rest would be preventable with a little care and thought (and some better research).

Most people recognise the damage that other doctors can do but like to think that *their* doctor is an honourable exception. This is entirely understandable. After all, we all like to think that our relationship with our own doctor is special, and that we have chosen someone reliable and knowledgeable to look after us. We like to think of our doctor as a personal and family friend. We all need to put some trust in the health care professionals upon whom we rely when we are ill.

But it is just as dangerous to assume that *your* doctor is entirely safe, sensible, knowledgeable, competent and error free as it would be to assume that you do not need to take care when driving, on the spurious grounds that road accidents only ever affect other people.

I suspect that all readers of this book make some effort to ensure that the tyres on their cars have plenty of tread, that the brakes are in good, working condition, that they wear seat belts and so on. Everyone knows that motor cars can kill and so sensible individuals do what they can to protect themselves.

And yet more than four times as many people a year die as a result of medical 'accidents' as die as a result of road accidents. Put another way this means that your doctor is four times as likely to kill you as your car.

The underlying problem is that even good, kind, conscientious doctors – who are honest and honourable, who care about their work and who do their very best for their patients – can still make people ill. And can still kill people.

Many of the problems caused by doctors are a result of prescription drug consumption. When he writes out a prescription your doctor has to rely upon the honesty and integrity of the drug company making the product he is prescribing. And since most drug companies do not operate in an honest way that is a fundamental error of trust which can lead to many problems. You suffer from his trust in the drug company. To that you must add the fact that all patients are individual and different. A drug which has proved effective and safe when given to 99 or 999 patients may still prove dangerous and deadly when given to the 100th or the 1000th patient. Every patient who takes a drug – even a well tried drug – is participating in an experiment. Most doctors either do not understand this or they forget it in the heat of daily practice.

The bottom line is that however good your doctor is – and however much you may trust him or her – you must share the responsibility for your own health and you must know when to tell your doctor if you think that the treatment with which he or she is providing you could be causing problems.

Here are my tips designed to help you make sure that you get the best out of your doctor (and every other doctor who treats you) – and minimise your chances of being made ill by a doctor.

1. Take a positive interest in your own health

Patients used to hand over their health (and their lives) to their doctors – without ever questioning what was happening to them. That is a dangerous way to live. Patients who take an interest in their own health may sometimes feel that the doctors and nurses who are looking after them regard them as a nuisance. But all the evidence shows that such patients get better quicker, suffer fewer unpleasant side effects and live longer than patients who simply lie back and allow the professionals to take over. If your doctor wants you to take a drug (and all tablets, capsules, medicines, potions, creams and so on are drugs) make sure you know what to expect. If your doctor wants you to have surgery then make sure that you know what the surgery entails, what the possible consequences might be and what the alternatives are. Good questions to ask your doctor are: 'Would you have this operation if you were me?' or: 'Would you recommend this operation to someone in your close family?'

2. Don't be afraid to ask for a second opinion

Many patients automatically trust their doctor – assuming that he or she must always be right. But that can be a deadly mistake.

It has always been diagnostic skills which have differentiated between the good doctor and the bad doctor. Treating sick people is easy. If you are a doctor and you know what is wrong with your patient you can look up the correct treatment in two minutes. Sadly, as I've shown earlier in this book, many doctors seem to have lost their abilities to diagnose accurately. And studies have shown that doctors are at their worst when dealing with patients with whom they feel uncomfortable. Narrow training means that doctors feel uncomfortable with a wide range of people. They often have difficulty relating to, talking to or acquiring information from people of different races, sexes or social backgrounds.

An even bigger problem is the fact that modern doctors rely far too much on technology – and far too little on building up any diagnostic skills of their own.

Old-fashioned doctors used to rely on what their patients told them and on what their own eyes, ears, noses and fingertips told them. Most important of all, perhaps, was the sixth sense that doctors used to acquire through years of clinical experience.

Modern doctors rely too much upon equipment which is often faulty, frequently badly calibrated and more often than not downright misleading.

So, the lesson here is a very simple one: do not automatically assume that your doctor's diagnosis must be right. If you are at all unhappy about the diagnosis – and feel that your doctor could be wrong – insist on a second opinion.

Telling your doctor that you want a second opinion will probably take a great deal of courage. Many doctors are sensitive creatures – they may show their hurt if their all-knowingness is questioned. But just remember that the stakes are high. Your life is at risk.

Finally, if there is time, don't be afraid to check out the past record of the doctor who is going to treat you. One surgeon working in a hospital may have a survival rate which is twice as good as another surgeon working in the same hospital. If you allow the less competent surgeon to operate on you then your chances of walking out of the hospital may be halved. Those are odds you cannot and should not ignore.

3. Remember Coleman's First Law of Medicine

If you develop new symptoms while receiving medical treatment then the chances are that the new symptoms are caused by the treatment you are receiving. Doctors do not like accepting that the treatments they recommend can do harm. It reminds them that they are mortal and fallible. But don't just ignore it if you develop a rash, indigestion, tinnitus, a headache or some other possible side effect: report it to your doctor straight away. Don't stop medication without asking his advice first. Some side effects are mild, and if the drug is working and helping to control or defeat a serious or life threatening condition, then the side effects may be of little consequence. But other side effects may kill. Many of the thousands who die each year might still be alive if they had taken action earlier while taking prescription drugs when side effects started. Remember, doctors are notoriously reluctant to admit that their therapy could be making you ill. This is partly through ignorance (doctors don't often bother to read drug company information sheets); partly through a fear of litigation (the doctor may be frightened that if he admits that his treatment has made you ill he will receive a letter from your lawyer), and partly through a natural human unwillingness to admit responsibility for something that has gone wrong (this brand of unwillingness is unusually well developed among doctors who are encouraged to think of themselves as godlike by many of their more passive patients).

4. Study all the options

In the chapter on holistic medicine I explained that there are very few truly holistic practitioners around. But there is nothing to stop you being a holistic patient. For example, if your doctor tells you that you need surgery ask him how long you have got before you need to make a decision – and then use that time to make sure that you assess all the possible options. When you are trying to choose between orthodox medicine, acupuncture, homoeopathy, osteopathy or whatever make a list of all the advantages and disadvantages of every available type of therapy – and every available practitioner. Look at the claims and the potential side effects of each therapy and ask each practitioner to tell you where you can find out more. Never forget that you are unique – and that your condition requires a unique solution.

91

5. Constantly acquire information

Information is the key to success in any field. If you want to be a successful investor then you need access to good information. You must know where to obtain information and you must know how to understand it. Exactly the same is true of health. In order to stay healthy – and regain good health if you fall ill – you must have access to good information. Only when you have the best information will you know what questions to ask and how to understand the answers. Doctors (and indeed many others in the health business) are notoriously bad at communicating – even though doctor-patient communication is of vital importance. Since doctors don't seem keen to bridge the understanding gap between patients and themselves it is up to you to make the effort. If you have a long term health problem then learn as much as you can about the disorder and all the possible types of treatment available. I have met patients with chronic health disorders (such as diabetes, arthritis, high blood pressure and so on) who know more about their condition than their doctors. Which patients do you think do best – those who know a great deal about their condition or those who know next to nothing?

6. Doctors often prescribe two drugs which interact dangerously.

If you're taking one drug and a doctor prescribes another – ask if the combination is really safe.

7. They may think you're someone else and treat you for the wrong disease.

If you don't want them to chop off the wrong leg or treat you for a prostate problem when you've really got a breast disorder make sure your doctor knows your name – and has the correct medical records when he decides on treatment.

8. Doctors prescribe unnecessarily.

Make it clear that you are happy to leave the surgery or clinic without a drug if you don't really need one. Most of the drugs prescribed today are unnecessary.

9. Doctors (particularly those working in hospitals) frequently order unnecessary tests.

Tests can often cause problems of their own. They can sometimes kill. Ask if a test will affect the treatment you receive. If it won't then what's the point of having the test? And read the chapter in this book on tests and investigations.

Chapter Seven

Why Women Live Longer Than Men

Women in developed countries can, on average, currently expect to live up to ten years longer than men.

That's a fact.

The oldest person in recorded history was a woman, Mme Jeanne Calment, who died at the age of 122 in 1997.

That's a fact.

Nine times as many women as men live to celebrate their one hundredth birthday.

That's a fact.

Men aged 55 to 64 are twice as likely as women of the same age to die from accidents or heart disease and four times as likely to commit suicide.

That's a fact.

It is widely believed that women live longer than men because of some genetic superiority. Indeed, most people believe that women have always lived longer than men.

Those are myths.

Up until the early part of the twentieth century life expectancy for men was pretty much the same as life expectancy for women; the difference only developed later during the twentieth century.

And I believe that the difference can be easily explained. The fact that women now live longer than men has nothing whatsoever to do with genetics or hormones. It is all down to lifestyle.

Here are the reasons why men now tend to die sooner than women.

1. For most of the twentieth century the average man pushed himself much harder than the average woman did. There were exceptions among both sexes, of course, but on the whole men felt that they had to

drive themselves hard in order to 'succeed'. (The definition of 'success' has varied from community to community.) The resultant high stress levels have helped produce a high incidence of heart disease and have damaged the immune systems of millions of men – thereby making vast numbers of men exceptionally vulnerable to many diseases including many varieties of cancer.

2. Smoking has, for decades, been very much a 'male' habit. For most of the twentieth century the number of male smokers far exceeded the number of female smokers. It was the popularity of smoking among men which partly explained the higher incidence of heart disease and some common cancers among men.

3. Throughout the twentieth century men were more likely to eat too much and more likely to eat the wrong (often high fat content) foods. Women have tended to be more conscious of the advantages of healthy eating than have men. In addition, women have traditionally been much more conscious of their size than have men and slimming clubs have always been more popular with women than with men.

4. For the first three quarters of the twentieth century most of the financial worries within a marriage were shouldered by the man. Many women never saw their husband's pay packet or bank details. A remarkable number of women never even knew how much their husbands earned. Worrying about money is one of the commonest stresses – and is particularly likely to result in ill health.

5. Generally speaking men have been woefully unwilling to be on the look out for – and aware – of abnormalities affecting their bodies. For decades women have routinely examined their own bodies – looking for abnormalities or early signs of developing disease. Men, on the other hand, have traditionally been unwilling to do this. Vast amounts of money have been spent teaching women how to examine their own breasts (in order to spot breast cancer). Virtually nothing has been spent teaching men how to examine their testicles (in order to spot cancer of the testes).

Women have been much more enthusiastic about learning the rudiments of self-help. Far more women than men are knowledgeable about alternative medicine. In addition, women have learnt to be more willing to seek help from a health care professional when they have found symptoms or signs which might indicate an underlying health problem. Why are so many women so much more comfortable about seeking medical advice than men? I suspect the explanation is simple. Women who get pregnant are accustomed to seeking medical help during their pregnant years. And it is usually the mother (rather than the father) who takes sick children along to the doctor's surgery.

6. Doctors are a major cause of sickness in our modern society but there are times when their help can be life-saving. And the sooner an individual seeks medical advice the greater likelihood that the doctor can deal with the problem satisfactorily.

   To all this must be added the fact that doctors have, for years, concentrated medical resources on health problems exclusively affecting women (such as cervical cancer and breast cancer) and virtually ignored health problems (such as prostate cancer) exclusively affecting men.

7. Alcohol was, for most of the twentieth century, a 'man thing'. Alcoholism – and alcohol induced damage – used to be much commoner among men than women. The female body is more susceptible to alcohol but excessive drinking has traditionally been something much more likely to affect men than women.

8. Workaholism was almost exclusively a male problem for the greater part of the twentieth century. Driven by ambition, competitiveness and a need to succeed millions of men pushed themselves to the limit and beyond. Many men have died – or become chronic invalids – because of their workaholism.

9. Throughout the twentieth century men have, generally speaking, been unwilling to talk to anyone about their problems. A man may joke with his best friend, or talk to him about his boss, his favourite football team or his car, but he is unlikely to open his heart, or to be prepared to share his innermost feelings. The average woman, on the other hand, does not have so much difficulty in opening up her heart and sharing her fears, hopes and aspirations with her best friend. Sharing personal fears is a good way of reducing the damage fears can do. The average man bottles up his fears and his worries – allowing those fears and worries to do a great deal of damage. By sharing her fears the average woman dramatically reduces the damage that is done.

10. When men take exercise it tends to be physically combative and potentially damaging. Football, for example, is likely to result in all sorts of physical injuries. The exercise men take also tends to be competitive in nature. So, for example, when men play golf or squash they are often determined to win. The result of all this is that when men take exercise it is likely to prove physically and mentally damaging. Feminine types of activity, on the other hand, tend to be gentler and less competitive. Women attend keep fit classes or aerobic classes, or go dancing. They benefit from their exercise programmes.

Chapter Eight

Why Women Won't Live Longer Than Men In The Future

The difference in life expectation between men and women will not continue far into the twenty-first century. This is not because men are going to live longer but because women are going to die sooner.

I base this prediction on these simple observations:

1. The number of women who smoke cigarettes is rising dramatically. Visit any large town, find yourself a convenient seat, and watch the young people go by. You will soon notice that smoking is now much commoner among young girls than it is among young boys. The statistical evidence supports this simple observation.

2. The incidence of alcoholism among women is rising too. A few decades ago it was rare to find a woman who had wrecked her life and her health with alcohol. Today it is commonplace.

3. Increasing numbers of women have been suckered by the women's liberation movement into believing that they owe it to themselves and their 'sisters' to take a more masculine attitude to life. It is common these days to find women in positions of managerial power. Modern women have demanded, and have taken, the same sort of damaging stresses as were endured by men throughout the twentieth century. Many women seem more aggressive and more 'masculine' than men. The incidence of stress related disorders among women is going to rocket in the next generation or two.

4. Women are taking their exercise more seriously – they have become more competitive and they push themselves harder when they are allegedly relaxing.

5. As women take an increasingly masculine approach to life so they aban-

96

don their traditional, health giving relationships with their female friends.
Many women now feel that it is somehow 'beneath them' to need to
share their fears, their feelings and their weak moments with other
women. Women are making themselves tougher and more self-suffi-
cient. The effect on their health will be bad.

Chapter Nine

Could Men Live As Long As Women?

In the next few decades we will see a dramatic fall in the difference between male and female life expectancies.

This will come about not because men are living longer but because women are dying earlier.

However, men could live longer if they chose to.

Here are my tips for any man wanting to live longer:

1. Don't smoke. Don't share a home or an office with anyone who smokes. Sit in no-smoking compartments and eat in restaurants which ban smoking. Few things are more deadly than tobacco smoke.

2. Learn to be aware of your body. If you notice a change do not delay but visit your doctor straight away.

3. Learn as much as you can about health care. Know how to treat yourself. If you have a specific health problem read books about it – so that you know as much as possible about the problem affecting your health. Be prepared to seek medical help if you need it – however inconvenient or embarrassing it might be.

4. Take regular, gentle, non competitive exercise. Don't push yourself too hard when exercising.

5. Learn to share your fears, your hopes, your disappointments, your ambitions and your feelings in general. Find a friend to whom you can talk about your most innermost thoughts. For most men the best and most sympathetic listener will be a woman rather than another man. Learn to talk to your wife or your partner, and don't be afraid to open your heart and share your feelings. It may be a cliché but it is often true to say that a worry shared is a worry halved.

6. Drink alcohol in moderation. One or two glasses of wine a day might well help you stay healthy. More may kill you.

7. Get a life. Find interests outside your work. Don't allow yourself to be suckered into putting all your energy into earning money. Relatively few workaholics get rich. But many workaholics die young.
8. Learn to eat in a healthy way. Eat more fruit and vegetables. Cut out meat. Avoid fatty foods.
9. Learn to relax. Learn to rest. Take time out. Give your body a chance to recover from the daily grind.

Chapter Ten

You *Can* Change Your Destiny!

Good health runs in families and if you can trace a long line of octogenarians in your family tree then you have also got a better than average chance of living to be eighty. Poor health runs in families, too, and if your parents and grandparents all died in their fifties and early sixties then I am afraid that doesn't augur well for your chances of celebrating your hundredth birthday – unless you are prepared to change your lifestyle to keep yourself healthy.

If you have a family history of any one of those diseases known to be transmitted genetically then you can help yourself by keeping an eye open for early signs or symptoms which might suggest that you too could become a victim. With almost all inherited diseases, making an early diagnosis is a vital step in preventing serious problems developing. If you know what to look for, and you watch and listen with care, you can do a great deal to reduce your risks and improve your life expectancy. And you may even be able to prevent the earliest of warning signs from developing simply by adapting your lifestyle.

The list which follows deals with some of the commonest inherited disorders. Remember that protecting yourself really is very much a case of being aware – and being prepared to change your lifestyle. For example, if other members of your family suffer from alcoholism then knowing that this problem may be inherited should give you an extra incentive to take care – and to make sure that your own drinking does not get out of hand.

Alcoholism

Risk rate: not known
Early symptoms: heavy drinking, comfort drinking
Action guide: drink warily

Allergy problems

Risk rate: up to 50% when one parent is affected, higher if both parents are affected
Early symptoms: vary; may include skin symptoms, wheezing, hay fever
Action guide: seek medical advice for any suggestive early symptom – be on the look out for possible allergens and then avoid them

Arthritis

Risk rate: not known
Early symptoms: aching, swollen joints
Action guide: lose excess weight, go on a vegetarian diet, rest when joints are swollen, hot or painful

Asthma

Risk rate: about 10% if one or both parents are affected (that is ten times the normal risk)
Early symptoms: wheezing, breathlessness
Action guide: don't smoke, keep out of smoky atmospheres, learn how to relax

Baldness

Risk rate: the risk among men increases according to the number of bald, male relatives
Early symptoms: loss of hair, usually in the 20s and early 30s
Action guide: be prepared to go bald with pride

Blindness

Risk rate: depends on the type of blindness
Early symptoms: partial or complete, temporary or permanent loss of vision
Action guide: seek immediate advice from an ophthalmologist

Cancer

Risk rate: varies enormously, but when several members of one family suffer from the same type of cancer professional advice should be sought
Early symptoms: vary with the type of cancer
Action guide: be generally watchful for early warning signs of cancer. Many cancers are curable – especially if caught early. Here are some of the cancer signs you should watch out for:

- Cancer of the large bowel: change in bowel habits (diarrhoea or constipation), unexplained weight loss, pain, passing blood
- Cancer of the cervix: unexplained bleeding or discharge, pain or bleeding after sex, weight loss
- Cancer of the breast: swelling or lump in breast, bloody discharge from nipple, enlarged glands in armpit, dimpling of the skin of the breast
- Cancer of the lung: persistent bad cough; blood in sputum, chest pain, wheezing, weight loss
- Cancer of the stomach: weight loss, persistent indigestion, vomiting blood, lump in abdomen, feeling full after very small meals
- Cancer of the liver: pain in abdomen, loss of appetite, weight loss, yellow eyes and skin, abdomen swollen
- Cancer of the ovary: irregular periods, hard lump in abdomen, pain during sex, bowel problems, excessive hair growth, voice gets deeper
- Cancer of the brain: headaches, vomiting, visual disturbances, weakness or paralysis, dizziness, fits, memory loss, personality changes
- Cancer of the skin: skin lesion that doesn't heal, bleeds, gets larger, changes shape, size or colour
- Cancer of the prostate: pain, urine retention, difficulty in passing urine
- Cancer of the testicle: change or swelling in testicle
- Cancer of the blood (leukaemia): tiredness, paleness, bruising, bleeding easily, lots of infections
- Cancer of the womb: bleeding after sex, lump felt in abdomen
- Cancer of the throat: hoarseness, lump in throat, difficulty in swallowing, swollen glands in neck

Remember: a patient with cancer may suffer from one, all or none of these symptoms. These symptom lists are not comprehensive. Patients may suffer from one or more of these symptoms without suffering from cancer. If you are at all worried see your doctor as soon as possible for advice.

Coronary heart disease

Risk rate: varies enormously but coronary heart disease is definitely an inherited disease
Early symptoms: chest pains and breathlessness
Action guide: don't smoke, don't allow yourself to become overweight, avoid excess stress, eat a low fat diet, take regular, gentle exercise

Diabetes

Risk rate: increased risk if one parent or sibling affected, higher risk if both parents are affected
Early symptoms: excessive thirst, frequent passing of urine, weight loss, boils
Action guide: don't get overweight, limit intake of sugar

Glaucoma

Risk rate: approximately 10% risk for brothers, sisters and children of sufferers
Early symptoms: visual problems and pain in or around the eye
Action guide: annual testing helps spot the disease early in those with a family history of glaucoma

High blood pressure

Risk rate: not known
Early symptoms: there often aren't any
Action guide: don't get overweight, avoid eating meat and fatty food, avoid unnecessary stress, learn to relax, do not smoke, have blood pressure taken regularly (or learn to take it yourself)

Migraine

Risk rate: general risk rate is 5%-10%, but this rises to 45% if one parent is affected and 70% if both parents are affected
Early symptoms: severe headaches, accompanied by nausea, vomiting and visual disturbances
Action guide: controlling stress can help minimise symptoms; migraine attacks are sometimes related to specific foodstuffs.

Peptic ulceration (stomach ulcer, duodenal ulcer)

Risk rate: when there is a family history, about 10% for men and 5% for women
Early symptoms: indigestion type pains, gastritis, nausea etc.
Action guide: eat regular meals, avoid excess alcohol, don't smoke, avoid excess stress, visit physician if early signs develop

Chapter Eleven

Reach 100 And Remain Alert And Active
(Tips To Help You Stay Young)

Our bodies age not from overuse but from disuse. The abuse to which we subject our various organs doesn't help. Most of us don't wear out. We rust away.

It's a myth to assume that growing old inevitably means growing ill. Raised blood pressure is not an inevitable consequence of ageing. Middle age spread isn't inevitable. You don't have to suffer with indigestion or hardening of the arteries just because you're getting older. Wrinkles aren't an inevitable consequence of ageing. Memory failure doesn't always affect everyone over the age of fifty. Sex drive doesn't necessarily falter with age.

It is widely assumed by our youth-obsessed society that anyone who struggles past their eightieth birthday must, by that time, be incontinent, incapable and incoherent. The elderly are widely regarded as inconsequential and insignificant in social and political terms. Doctors generally expect that ageing will inevitably produce an unending series of physical, mental and emotional problems. The elderly are expected to lose their memory, their bone strength, their muscles, their creativity and just about everything else which makes life worth living. Not long ago a senior politician in the US announced that the terminally ill elderly have a 'duty to die and get out of the way'.

In an attempt to help you fend off this awful fate, the charlatans will make you all sorts of promises. Take a pinch of that and a teaspoonful of this and it will be like having a portrait of Dorian Gray in the attic. So they say. Don't believe a word of it. The 'anti-ageing' business is the medical equivalent of the time-share industry. The 'keep you young with wonder pills' industry claimed that one group of country folk routinely live to be

100, thanks to their drinking water. Investors had bought land near the 'fountain of youth' before this was exposed as a hoax. A village in the USSR was widely promoted as a breeding ground for centenarians. This was nonsense. The villagers had altered their birth records to escape conscription into the army.

Most signs of ageing develop as a result of bad habits more than anything else. Plenty of centenarians are lively, productive, alert and active. They do not associate old age with dependence. They refuse to accept that age necessarily brings limitations. They fight for the things that matter but ignore the problems that don't. They know that skills don't have to deteriorate with age. They know that doctors who say things like 'At your age, what can you expect?' are ignorant fools who should be doing something else for a living.

Some people age better than others. Why?

Are there secrets to successful ageing? Of course there are.

So, here's what you can do to keep yourself looking, feeling and acting younger. Follow this recipe and you'll dramatically extend your potential life-span. (Though I do not, of course, guarantee that you won't be run over by a bus or struck by lightning.) There are no miracle answers. You have to work at staying young. But if you follow the advice here – and change your life to match the information I've collected for you – your body and your mind will be much better equipped to fight the factors which lead to the signs of ageing. And these relatively insignificant sounding changes can result in a dramatic improvement in life expectation. Just cleaning your teeth properly can add years to your life. Keeping your immune system in good shape can help to protect you from an enormous range of potentially deadly diseases. Choosing a piece of fruit instead of another burger won't add years to your life but regularly choosing fruit instead of burgers will add years to your life. It's remarkably easy to add five to ten years to your life expectation – just by making simple lifestyle changes. It is only slightly more difficult to add an extra five years to that. The 40-year-old who does average things with his or her life will have the average life expectation of a 40-year-old. The 40-year-old who lives an unhealthy lifestyle may be physiologically equivalent to a 50-year-old. And the 40-year-old who lives wisely may have the body of a 30-year-old.

1. Eat wisely

One third of all cancers are caused by eating the wrong foods. Many cases of heart disease are food related too.

To live a long, healthy life you should avoid red meat. Red meat consumption is a major risk factor for colon cancer and prostate cancer. You should also keep your consumption of fat down to around 15% of your total calorie intake (rather than the 30% currently recommended by government experts everywhere) and eat plenty of fruits, vegetables, grains and legumes. Cut down on sweets (puddings), avoid processed foods and use olive oil rather than animal fat and butter. Avoid hydrogenated fats as well as animal fats such as butter and cheese. Hydrogenated fats are commonly used in the manufacture of biscuits, cakes and white bread and dramatically increase the risk of heart disease. Most fast food restaurants cook with hydrogenated vegetable oil and serve food which is high in fat, cholesterol and sugar. Fast food, fast death. And packaged foods which don't need to be stored in the freezer are usually high in fat and sugar too. Cut your intake of saturated fat and you'll probably live longer.

Men should eat regular servings of tomato paste and tomato products. The carotenoid found in tomatoes (lycopene) will, when heated and eaten with oil, provide an immune strengthening anti-oxidant that helps reduce the risk of prostate cancer developing. Raw tomatoes and tomato juice aren't a great help. The lycopene seems to release most effectively through cooking. And the presence of oil seems to be necessary for the lycopene to be absorbed. The tomato sauce on pizza is excellent, but pizza often (though not always) contains cheese which is usually high in saturated fats. Better ways to get the lycopene-rich tomato products are to eat tomato sauces on pasta or tomato-based soups. Alternatively, even putting tomato ketchup onto other foods may help.

At least two thirds of your daily calorie intake should be in the form of complex carbohydrates – including fresh fruit and vegetables, potatoes, rice, pasta and wholegrain breads and cereals. Keep your intake of protein to between 10% and 20% of your daily diet. Too much protein in the diet can put pressure on the kidneys (which deteriorate with age). You don't need a high protein intake to build up muscle strength.

2. Watch your calorie intake
Remember that our calorie needs fall as we age. At the age of 20 men can usually eat 3,000 calories a day and women can usually eat 2,200 calories a day without putting on any weight. But by the age of 80 men need only about 2,400 calories while women need only 1,600 calories. Reducing your calorie intake will probably help you lose weight – as well as keep your weight under control. Remember that the best way to lose weight permanently is to change your eating habits. Clever, short term crash diets rarely produce the long term results that people hope for.

3. Give up meals completely
Eating three square meals a day is old-fashioned and bad for you. Mealtimes are not natural. They were invented because they just happen to fit in

with the way most of us work and live. If you get most of your calories three times a day at fixed meal times then you are almost certain to end up over-weight. Calories that aren't burnt up straight away will end up stuck on your hips. In addition, there is also no doubt that you will make yourself more prone to stomach problems. Regular meals are better for you than irregular meals and regular small meals are better than regular big meals. By eating regularly you'll be helping to mop up some of the acid in your stomach. If you eat irregularly the acid in your stomach will have nothing to get its teeth into.

We've lost the art of knowing when we've had enough to eat. Most of us make the mistake of always finishing the food on our plates because we've been trained that wasting food is wrong.

You will be much healthier if you re-establish control of your appetite control centre by eating when you feel hungry, stopping when you feel full (or better still, just before you feel full) – and nibbling smaller meals more frequently rather than stuffing yourself with large meals occasionally.

The healthy way to eat is to eat mini-meals – and to eat little and often. You probably think of it as nibbling. Marketing experts call it 'graz-ing' because it is the way that wild animals eat. Whatever you call it eating numerous small meals is much better for you – in a number of ways – than eating just three big meals.

4. Make sure you get enough sleep

Don't try to survive on five hours sleep a night. You will suffer. Men need eight hours of sleep a night. Women need seven hours of sleep a night.

5. Take regular exercise

One of the main reasons why life expectation is not as good as it should be (and why so many people are disabled and crippled) is that most of us take far too little exercise. We travel everywhere by car or public transport. We use lifts instead of walking up the stairs. Our homes are filled with labour-saving devices such as washing machines, vacuum cleaners and tumble driers.

What sort of exercise do you need?

Regular and gentle are the two key words.

Regular exercise can help prevent or delay diabetes, obesity and heart disease. Regular exercise helps keep your weight under control, helps pre-vent osteoporosis and helps boost your immune system – which helps to prevent cancer. Prostate cancer and breast cancer are both less likely to occur in individuals who exercise regularly. Women who exercise for four hours a week have a 60% reduction in breast cancer risk. Just fifteen to thirty minutes of walking or cycling a day is probably enough to produce a significant reduction in cancer risk. But most adults take little or no exercise. People who are sedentary lose around 30% of their strength and a third of their muscle mass between the ages of 20 and 70. This loss is largely a result of lack of exercise.

Swimming, walking, cycling and dancing are all excellent forms of exercise which help to get rid of unwanted fat and to improve the effectiveness of the heart. But you need to do resistance exercises – such as weight training – in order to prevent the loss of muscle tissue. It is worth remembering that increasing muscle mass helps by improving the body's ability to burn fat. Resistance exercise will help your body get rid of excess weight.

Remember that before beginning an exercise programme you should consult your doctor – and, ideally, have a medical examination. Visit a local gym and find a qualified expert to help advise you before you start an exercise programme.

6. Live within your means
Learn to manage your finances so that you live within your means. If possible, try to make sure that you have a little money put to one side for emergencies. Knowing that your nest egg is there will give you greater confidence and help to reduce stresses which are related to money.

7. Protect your hearing
Loud noises that make you feel uncomfortable can damage your hearing. A refrigerator hums at about 40 decibels. Normal conversation is usually conducted at around 60 decibels. City traffic makes a noise of about 80 decibels. Fireworks, motorcycles, music at concerts or listened to through headphones, may all produce between 120 and 140 decibels. Anything above 75 decibels can produce hearing loss. Limit your exposure to unnecessary noises and use ear plugs whenever you have to be in the vicinity of something very noisy. If you don't your hearing will probably be permanently damaged.

8. Watch your blood pressure
Even a modest rise (10 mm or so) in blood pressure can result in a significant (10%) increase in the risk of serious damage. To begin with blood pressure goes up without symptoms. Have your blood pressure checked annually. And take action to keep your blood pressure under control. (Do not smoke, do not put on excess weight, keep your intake of fatty foods down, do not expose yourself to unnecessary stresses, learn to relax etc.).

9. Beware of drugs which can cause 'senility'
You don't have to lose your mind just because there are more candles on your birthday cake than there used to be. Doctors used to classify all elderly people as 'senile' until proved otherwise. Then the phrase 'organic brain

syndrome' became fashionable. And doctors began to expect every individual over the age of seventy to be suffering from 'dementia'.

These days Alzheimer's disease is the fashionable diagnosis. But it simply isn't true that every elderly person must inevitably become senile or demented or a victim of Alzheimer's disease. And even when an elderly individual does develop symptoms of dementia it isn't necessarily the case that the condition is incurable. Infections can cause dementia like symptoms. As can small strokes. But the commonest cause of treatable dementia among the elderly is undoubtedly doctor induced: side effects associated with prescription drugs are a significant cause of apparent senility. When the drugs are stopped the symptoms will disappear.

You should not, of course, ever just stop a drug that has been prescribed by a doctor. You need to talk to the doctor first.

10. Exercise your brain – use it or lose it

There is no point in maintaining a healthy body if you lose your mind. Studies have shown that if you are going to survive into (and enjoy) a genuine old age you need to retain the ability to plan your life, to start new tasks and to see them through.

Your brain has plenty of spare capacity. You have to lose quite a high percentage of the neurones in a certain area before you start to notice any problems. And you can delay the onset of problems – and help to improve the situation when problems have developed – by deliberately doing whatever you can to increase the number of new dendrites in your brain.

Dendrites are the finger-like extensions which connect neurones together – and which allow neurones to exchange chemical and electrical messages. The cells you have in your brain can grow new dendrites. Sometimes new dendrites can grow to replace existing connections. Sometimes they can grow to help provide more space for messages that can't get through. And sometimes they create entirely new connections with other neurones.

So how can you stimulate the number of dendrites in your brain?

Simple. You use your brain as much as you can.

When you take up a new interest or learn a new skill your brain will form new dendrites. The extent of the formal education you have seems to be irrelevant but there is good evidence to support the theory that the more active you keep your mind the less likely you will be to develop any variety of dementia. Take up a challenging mental activity (such as learning to play a musical instrument, learning to paint, writing, sculpting, learning a language) and you will be giving your brain exercise that will keep it healthy. You can even help yourself by doing puzzles and games. Playing chess or bridge and doing jigsaw puzzles or crossword puzzles will all help to keep your mind in shape. Learning stimulates the growth of new dendrites and creates more effective brain power. The more complex the activity the better the workout.

(Learning and practising a musical instrument is particularly useful since it requires coordinating different parts of the brain and involves reading, listening, memorising, performing fairly complicated physical manoeuvres and having new ideas. This sort of activity means that links between different parts of the brain are strengthened. If you learn musical pieces which bring back good memories than you can also use music to help you combat stress.) See Chapter Thirteen for more advice on how to increase your brain power.

11. Change your personality so that you feel happier

Our personalities usually remain fairly stable after the age of twenty. There tend not to be any major changes. But as we become older we tend to become more like ourselves. The shy and reclusive become more shy and more reclusive. The irritable and edgy become more irritable and more edgy. Studies of centenarians have shown that people who live a long time tend to be able to maintain their emotional focus and to be able to concentrate on surviving. Personality is one of the most important factors in survival and longevity is a result not of avoiding stressful circumstances but of having responded to stress in an effective and constructive way. People who have a positive way of looking at things, and who can maintain inwardly relatively calm in the face of crises, are much more likely to stay healthy and live longer. Your personality can have as big an impact on your longevity as your genes, your immune system or your cardiovascular system.

A study which followed a group of American schoolchildren for more than 70 years found that individuals who were dependable and conscientious were more likely to live longer. People – especially men – who were prudent, truthful and free of vanity were 30% less likely to die in any given year than those who did not have these qualities. It is, it seems, these particular traits which lead to a healthy old age.

The one quality which counters against longevity is neuroticism. Neuroticism is usually defined as an extra susceptibility to anger, sadness, fear and guilt – all of which can lead to anxiety, hostility, self consciousness and depression – and there seems no doubt that these are unhealthy personality traits.

Anxieties and fears can have a negative impact on health and life expectation and individuals who are prone to worry are less capable of adapting to, and coping with, unfamiliar or threatening situations. Those who suffer a great deal from anxiety are more likely to have disturbed immune systems or irregular heart beats – and they are, as a direct consequence, more likely to have a heart attack.

When the body is switched onto alert (as happens with individuals who are unusually susceptible to stress) the hormones produced can affect just about every part of the body. Individuals who can remain calm in a crisis and who are less prone to unrealistic thinking are, inevitably, far more flexible and far more adaptable. Emotional stress causes ageing and learning how to cope with stress is a vital factor in living a long, healthy life.

(An additional reason why stress susceptibility causes health problems is that neurotic individuals who are exceptionally susceptible to stress are more likely to use aids such as tobacco or alcohol to help them cope.)

We cannot change our basic personalities. But we can change the way in which we respond to situations. Ambitious, hard working individuals probably cannot change their basic attitudes towards life but they can avoid unnecessary stressful situations, they can spend more time doing things which they find enjoyable and relaxing, and they can learn to cope more effectively with new situations and with unavoidable stresses.

12. He who laughs longest lasts longest

A good sense of humour is known to be associated with better physical health and with a strong mental approach to life. Humour is one of the best 'coping' mechanisms we have. Humour can help us deal with life's many hard realities and it can help us deal with sorrow and hurt. With humour in our lives we are better able to cope emotionally and better able to think creatively. Humour can turn embarrassing situations into hilarious anecdotes.

Smiling and laughing give the body the same sort of benefits as exercise such as walking or swimming – indeed, laughter has been described as 'internal jogging'.

Laughing increases the amount of oxygen inhaled and the amount of carbon dioxide exhaled; it also increases the blood pressure just enough to give the tissues extra supplies of oxygen and it gives the heart essential exercise too. Paradoxically, laughter helps promote both alertness and a feeling of being relaxed; it makes muscles tense and then relaxes and stimulates the release of neurotransmitters which improve the functioning of the brain. Laughter also improves the effectiveness of the immune system and helps reduce anxiety and tension.

13. Lose any excess weight – and keep it off

Eight out of ten centenarians say that their current weight is close to what it was when they were young adults. Most of us in the Western world eat far too much food – and far too much of the wrong types of food. Overweight is one of the most significant killers.

Research in Japan has shown that death rates from heart disease, stroke and cancer are between 31% and 41% lower among adults who eat fewer calories than are in a standard calorie-rich Western diet.

Another study, this time done in Holland, showed that non obese middle aged men who cut their calorie intake by a fifth for ten weeks had lower blood pressure and had lost 10% of their body weight. Obesity is linked to colon, rectal and prostate cancer in men and to cancers of the gallbladder, breast, cervix, uterus and ovaries in women. Men and women whose body weight is 40% greater than average for their height and age group are a third more likely to develop cancer than the general population. Remember that yo-yo dieting is bad for you. Lose weight slowly and steadily.

14. Avoid unnecessary stress
If you have three or more major life crises in a single year your health will be severely threatened. If you are planning to move house and change your job try to make sure that you are not exposed to any other major stresses in the same twelve month period. Don't try to lose weight at the same time as you are moving house. Don't even try to lose weight at the same time as you are giving up cigarettes or starting a new exercise programme. And try to minimise your exposure to minor, avoidable stresses.

15. Build up your resistance to stress
Having good friends to whom you can turn for support will dramatically improve your life expectancy. Learning strategies for coping with stress will also help enormously.

16. Keep your consumption of drugs to a minimum.
Before taking a prescription drug get your doctor to confirm that the drug is essential. Ask him what will happen to you if you don't take it. Remember that 40% of the people who take a prescription drug suffer unpleasant, noticeable or potentially lethal side effects. And remember too that one in six patients in hospital are there because they have been made ill by doctors. If you take 'repeat' prescriptions check regularly with your doctor that the drugs are essential. You should be equally cautious about taking over-the-counter non-prescription drugs. Remember that many governments now allow drug companies to sell powerful and potentially lethal drugs without a prescription. (Governments which run state health services do this to reduce their costs.) And be cautious too about taking alternative remedies. Taking responsibility for your own health means being cautious and constantly selective about the medicines you take – whatever their origin.

17. Look after your friends

People who have good and loyal friends are more likely to recover from a heart attack than people who have few or no friends. Amazingly, one study has shown that people with no friends at all are three times as likely to die as those with just one friend. A friendly face, a smile and a hug can lower the level of dangerous chemicals and increase the body's self-healing powers.

18. Don't turn your back on religious beliefs

Freud claimed that man invented God to use as a shield against the help-lessness of living in an endlessly hostile world. Whether he was right or not is irrelevant in health terms. Twenty years ago a study of nearly 1,500 people of 65 or more showed that individuals who attended church were healthier than those who didn't. Indeed, the survey showed that having a religious belief played a greater part in health satisfaction than any other factor (including smoking or alcohol use). Those who take comfort from religion are less likely to suffer pain and more likely to remain independent. Frequent prayer can lower blood pressure and reduce pain and church goers tend to have stronger immune systems than non churchgoers.

19. Learn to adapt – and be prepared for change

We live in a constantly changing world. Indeed our world now changes faster than at any other time in history. And the pace of general change is going to continue to increase. The individuals most likely to survive in our modern world are, inevitably, those who are most capable of adapting to all these changes; capable of controlling their own local environment, capable of taking charge of situations in which they find themselves and capable of finding a new way to do things. The adaptable individual will use a hearing aid or a walking stick rather than struggle on and put themselves at risk. The adaptable individual will say 'no' when necessary, will walk away from difficult situations when it makes sense to do so and will ask for help when they need it.

20. Come to terms with death

An ability to come to terms with one's own mortality is not defeatist. It is, on the contrary, sensible, practical and liberating to accept that death is eventually inevitable. Preparing for death does not mean giving up. It is something that we should all do on a regular basis – even though we might realistically hope and expect to have many years of healthy and profitable life ahead of us. Facing death without fear enables us to assess our life to date, to decide what mistakes we have made and to redirect our remaining years so that when our times comes we can, in the words of Plutarch, quit without regret.

21. Learn from your mistakes

Come to terms with – and forget – past mistakes. Learn from them and move on. Allowing yourself to grieve over errors and past injustices may destroy your present and devalue your future.

22. Don't worry about occasional memory lapses

Nearly seven out of ten adults are worried that they are losing their memory. Most people over the age of 30 complain of memory loss.

Occasional memory lapses are, however, quite normal. They occur naturally throughout life and they aren't a sign of developing dementia. Just because you can't quite find the word you want (even though you know it is on the tip of your tongue) you aren't necessarily showing the first signs of dementia or Alzheimer's disease.

23. Drink wisely

One single measure of alcohol a day may, it seems, help improve your health and longevity. (Men can have two small drinks. Women should limit themselves to one.) Any more than that will damage your health. Individuals who are at risk in any way (because of an addictive personality or any existing health problems, or because of a family history of alcohol abuse) should not follow this step but should avoid alcohol completely.

24. Learn to survive on the roads

Don't drink and drive a car or ride a motorcycle or a bicycle. Buckle your seat belt before you drive. Have a car fitted with airbags if possible – unless you are under five feet two inches tall or sit extremely close to the wheel. Never use a mobile phone while driving. Use as big a car as you can afford (bigger is slightly safer on the road) and have it maintained regularly by someone who knows what they are doing. Drive defensively.

25. Take care of your teeth and gums

Brush and floss your teeth regularly and visit a dentist and hygienist (both of whom you trust) regularly. Gingivitis and periodontal disease can cause tooth loss and can also affect your whole immune system and cause ageing. The bacteria that cause gum disease seem to trigger an immune response which causes general inflammation around the body – including the arteries. It is possible, therefore, that poor dental hygiene may lead to heart disease. Brushing and flossing can help you live longer. Dental cavities don't make much difference to your overall health or your life expectancy (though cavities may lead to a need for dentures and may, therefore, affect your ability to chew food properly) but gingivitis and similar diseases can cause serious, general problems. One survey showed that individuals who have gingivitis and periodontitis have a mortality rate that is up to 46% higher than those who don't. Gum disease can increase your chances of dying from heart disease, stroke or infection.

26. Avoid environmental carcinogens
Up to 15% of cancers are caused by carcinogens encountered at work. (For women this figure is rather lower). But the most significant environmental cause of cancer is tobacco smoke. Smoking can dramatically reduce your life expectancy. Lung cancer is still the commonest form of cancer. And most cases of lung cancer are caused by smoking. But lung cancer isn't the only type of cancer known to be linked to smoking. Colon cancer and cancers of the larynx, oesophagus, bladder, kidney and pancreas are all linked to tobacco smoking. Heart disease is much commoner among smokers too – as are digestive problems. Tobacco smoke will weaken your immune system.

However, the good news is that if you give up smoking you can pretty much restore your life expectancy to normal. There is an almost immediate positive effect and your body starts to recover within twelve hours of giving up smoking. Within a few months you should start to notice the improvement in your general health.

Passive smokers are damaged by tobacco smoke almost as much as smokers and the partners of smokers (who must, inevitably, end up breathing in tobacco smoke) have a dramatically increased risk of developing cancer and dying early. Spending one hour in a smoke-filled room is the equivalent of smoking four cigarettes.

Incidentally, it is a myth that smoking a cigar is safer than smoking a cigarette. Cigars are at least as dangerous – both for the smoker and the innocent bystander – as cigarettes. They produce carbon monoxide, hydrogen cyanide, ammonia and all sorts of other baddies.

27. Breathe clean air
Try to breathe clean air as often as you can. In cities air quality varies enormously from place to place. Try to live near a park, on a quiet road and, if you live in an apartment, above the ground floor. Remember that air pollution is often a problem indoors too. Building sickness is caused by poor indoor air quality. Air conditioning systems which simply re-circulate air result in the fact that if one person in the building has an infection the chances are that everyone in the building will soon have it. Buildings which do not have opening windows are particularly prone to cause problems. Air filtration systems really don't make much difference. If you get constant headaches, nausea and respiratory infections – and always feel tired – ask your fellow workers if they feel the same. If they do then the chances are that it is your building which is making you ill.

Living near to a busy road is bad for your health. Living on a corner or a junction or on a hill can all dramatically reduce the quality of the air your breathe.

Chemicals from diesel fumes are believed to cause 10,000 deaths a year in the UK – and 60,000 deaths a year in the US. Japanese researchers have discovered a compound in the exhaust emissions of diesel engines which, they claim, is the most carcinogenic substance ever analysed and is probably responsible for the high incidence of lung cancer among city dwellers. (This is not, however, the only carcinogen in diesel fumes).

The production of carcinogens increases dramatically when engines are pulling heavy loads. The obvious answer is to regulate the size of loads that diesel trucks can pull. Naturally, however, politicians are unlikely to risk annoying the transport industry by pushing for any changes.

The only practical answer is for you and I to do our best to avoid areas where diesel trucks congregate. The most dangerous spots are probably steep or long hills where truck engines will be under great strain.

28. Remember that most accidents aren't accidents at all
Eighty per cent of all accidents are avoidable.

29. Stay young with more sex
The more orgasms you have a year the younger you will feel, look and act. Mutually monogamous and safe sex can dramatically improve your life expectancy. Those who have satisfying sex every day will, all other things being equal, survive much longer than those who have sex once a week. A heterosexual relationship is more likely to lead to improved health and increased longevity than a homosexual relationship.

On the other hand unprotected sex with casual high risk partners (i.e. partners who are willing to have casual sex) is likely to lead to a reduction in life expectation. Remember that some sexually transmitted diseases do not cause any symptoms but may exist silently. Remember too that four out of ten individuals with serious sexually transmitted diseases admit to not telling their partners about their disease.

Regular sex (which you enjoy) can add nearly a decade to your life expectancy.

30. Beware of too much sunshine
Individuals who have red hair and fair skin are most at risk from the sun. Wear long-sleeved shirts or blouses and a hat and avoid going out in the sun when it isn't necessary. Sun bathing is one of the most extraordinary stupid things people do. Those who use sunbeds probably need certifying.

Your risk of developing skin cancer is largely determined by the amount of time you have been exposed to the sun. Sun exposure as a child or young adult is particularly potent. Individuals who were badly sunburnt as children are especially susceptible to skin cancer. Individuals with a family history of skin cancer, or who were badly sunburnt as children, should take extra care.

Look for changes in the shape, size or colour of moles. Any mole that is irregular, has variable colours or is more than a quarter of an inch across should be checked by a doctor. Get a friend to check parts of your body which you cannot examine yourself.

Remember that although cancers are most likely to occur on areas which have been sunburnt, too much sun can cause cancers elsewhere on the body. If you regularly work outside and have tanned arms and legs you are more likely to get skin cancer on white parts of your body.

Ten to fifteen minutes of sun a day on your face, neck, arms and hands should be enough to provide you with the necessary vitamin D your body needs. (Vitamin D helps to strengthen the immune system and helps to cut down your risk of developing certain types of cancer. If you don't get much sun you may need vitamin D in food or supplements – but it is vitally important to take care not to exceed the recommended intake of this vitamin.)

Chapter Twelve

Easy Steps You Can Take To Reduce Your Cancer Risk By 80%

Cancer is one of the biggest killers of our time. More than one in three people will some day hear a doctor say the dreaded words: 'I'm afraid you've got cancer'. (Within a few years the figure will be one in two.)

But despite all the research which has been done there are more myths and unjustified fears about this disease than any other disease in the world.

One myth is that this disease always kills. It doesn't. Between a third and a half of the people who get this disease recover – usually living long, perfectly healthy, perfectly normal lives.

But another, even more important, myth is that no one knows what causes this disease and as a result it is quite unavoidable.

That's a really dangerous myth because we now know a tremendous amount about what causes this disease. In fact we know what causes a staggering 80% of cancers.

It stands to reason, therefore, that if you want to cut your cancer risk by 80 % all you have to do is to try to avoid those things which are responsible.

'But surely,' someone said when I first mentioned this, 'if doctors know so much about the things which causes cancer we would have already heard about them – and been warned to avoid them by the government and the medical profession.'

Sadly, things aren't quite so straightforward these days.

I believe that the truth about the causes of cancer has been deliberately suppressed – by businessmen and politicians.

***

Here are my tips for healthy living. Follow these tips and you could cut your cancer risk by 80%.

1. Eat foods which will boost your immune system. In general, eat plenty of fruit, vegetables and seeds. Your chances of developing cancer – for example cancers of the lung, breast, colon, bladder, oral cavity, stomach and cervix – will go down if you eat plenty of vegetables. Fruit and vegetables contain plenty of fibre which can help to protect you against cancer – plus special anti-cancer ingredients. The best anti-cancer foods to eat include: apples, asparagus, baked beans, broccoli, Brussels sprouts, carrots, cauliflower, chick peas, corn, garlic, grapefruit, kidney beans, lentils, onions, oranges, pineapple, brown rice, soya beans, spinach and strawberries. There is a full list of recommended foods in my book *Superbody* (published by the European Medical Journal).

2. Keep your fat consumption down. Avoid foods which are rich in fat. Avoid dairy products. There is evidence linking fatty food to cancer – including cancers of the breast, prostate, uterus, ovary, pancreas, stomach and colon. Avoid butter, milk, cream and other fatty foods. Keep down your intake of vegetable fats too. Fat intake and breast cancer are closely linked. If you choose a high fat diet you are making a conscious decision to increase your risk of developing cancer.

3. Do not eat meat. Researchers have linked eating meat to cancer – including cancers of the breast, uterus, colon, rectum, pancreas and kidney. Red meat seems the most dangerous type of meat – beef, for example, has been specifically linked to colon cancer. Women who eat meat are significantly more likely to develop breast cancer than women who rarely or never consume meat. Several studies have shown a relationship between the incidence of prostate cancer and the consumption of meat. Smoked, barbecued, salt cured and salt pickled foods pose extra risks. If you don't want to get cancer – don't eat meat.

4. Prepare food carefully to preserve the vitamin and mineral content and to avoid the risk of infection.

5. Buy organic food whenever you can.

6. Do not drink unfiltered tap water.

7. Take a supplement rich in anti-oxidants.

8. Learn how to relax your mind and your body. And be prepared to spend a little time putting your learning into practice. Do your best to avoid unnecessary stresses.

9. Watch out for the early warning signs of cancer (such as unusual lumps, fresh bleeding, weight change etc.). And seek help straight away if you think you spot a warning sign.

10. Don't take drugs you don't really need. And be cautious about the prom-

ises made for vaccines. Try to keep away from hospitals, doctors' clinics and other places where sick people congregate (and where you are, consequently, likely to pick up new infections). Remember Coleman's First Law of Medicine: 'If you develop new symptoms while being treated for any medical condition the chances are that the new symptoms are caused by the treatment you are receiving.'

11. Try to avoid buildings which have closed circuit air conditioning or heating systems.

12. Avoid air travel whenever possible. Airlines tend to recirculate dirty air – thereby exposing passengers to many new (and potentially deadly) bugs.

13. If you have a mobile telephone use it sparingly – for emergencies rather than for idle chit-chat.

14. Don't cook with a microwave oven. (See my book *Food for Thought* for the reasons why.)

15. Don't have unnecessary X-rays. Routine X-rays are a possible threat to your health. Most X-rays are unnecessary. Check with your doctor that your X-ray is essential.

16. Control your weight. If you weigh just 22 pounds more than you did when you were 18 years old then you are probably at risk. Losing weight isn't just a matter of vanity. Women who are more than 40% overweight are 55% more likely to die of cancer – including cancers of the breast, uterus, ovary and gallbladder. Men who are more than 40% overweight are 33% more likely to die of cancer – with cancers of the colon, rectum and prostate among the cancers they risk developing.

17. Don't smoke and keep away from people who smoke. It isn't enough not to smoke yourself. You are also at risk if you spend too much time inhaling other people's tobacco smoke. For example, the World Health Organization has warned that: 'in marriages where one partner smokes and the other does not, the risk of lung cancer to the non-smoker is 20%-50% higher.' If you are travelling on public transport, eating in restaurants or going to the cinema choose non-smoking areas whenever possible.

18. Beware of sunshine. A little sunshine is good for you. But too much sunshine can cause skin cancer. Sunbathing is pointlessly reckless. Most cases of skin cancer are optional.

19. Beware of electrical appliances. Don't sit closer than three feet to your TV set. Unplug your electric blanket before getting into bed. Don't sit within two and a half or three feet of a VDU. Don't sit or stand too close to electrical appliances – electricity is almost certainly more dangerous than you think. Try not to live close to a power line or electricity sub-station.

20. Minimise your consumption of food additives. If you eat a lot of packaged foods you almost certainly eat too many food additives. The average individual eats around 5.5 lb. (2.5kg) of food additives every year. Food additives are potential hazards. You can minimise your consumption of food additives by eating a high proportion of fresh food.
21. Drink less alcohol. Alcohol can cause cancers of the mouth, larynx, oesophagus, stomach and pancreas. To minimise your cancer risk you should limit yourself to one or possibly two modest drinks a day.

Naturally, I cannot and do not guarantee that you won't get cancer if you follow my advice. But I do passionately believe that your chances of developing cancer will be significantly lower than it will be if you take no action to protect yourself.

Chapter Thirteen

Increase Your Mental Abilities With Age

Are you worried about losing your mental faculties as you age? Do you believe that your memory and ability to concentrate and think creatively must inevitably decline as you get older?

Forget those fears. They are based on myths.

If you know how to do it you can improve your brain power through your fifties, sixties, seventies, eighties and beyond.

Like many people I have for several decades believed the often re-peated assertion that every day we live we lose several million neurones – and that, consequently, our brains become steadily less agile and less capa-ble as the years go by.

The steady but relentless loss of neurones, I understood, explains why creativity falters as we age and why, for example, mathematicians are often said never to have any original ideas after the age of about twenty six.

I now believe that claim was no more than a well-established medical myth; given credibility and sustained simply through constant repetition rather than solid research.

Ask a doctor where this claim originated and you are likely to be re-ferred to another doctor or, perhaps, a book. Check with that doctor or book and you will be referred to another expert and another book. And so it goes on – with the myth going round and round in a never ending circle.

I haven't been able to find any solid research to support the conten-tion. I believe it is, like the age-old claim that taking vitamin E supplements will improve your sex life, just one of those mysterious medical myths.

And when you stop to think about it the myth is, indeed, quite non-sensical. There are around one thousand billion (a million million) brain cells or neurones in the average human brain. If we lost a million brain cells a day from the age of 20 the overall loss of brain cells would still be fairly insignificant a century later.

Research done at the University of California has confirmed that, in normal, healthy, active brains there is no loss of brain cells.

Other researchers, at the National Institute of Ageing in the US, have shown that an old human brain shows just as much metabolic activity – and is, therefore, just as active and as efficient – as a young human brain.

A 70-year-old brain uses just as much oxygen and has just as good a blood flow as a 20-year-old brain. If brains lost neurones they would need less oxygen and a reduced blood flow as they got older. The myth of neuronal decay with age is just that – a myth.

And yet it is partly this myth which has been – and is – responsible for many of the prejudices against the elderly.

Many men and women who are regarded as 'old' (but who may only be in their early 50s) are discovering that these prejudices result in forced early retirement, or in their being regarded by younger colleagues as irrelevant dinosaurs, incapable of originality and steeped in obstinacy.

***

The joyful truth is not only that your brain is not decaying as you live but that you can, if you wish, constantly improve the power of your brain (and this means your intelligence) as you get older – not by increasing the number of cells but by increasing the number of connections between the cells. You can, I repeat, improve your intelligence as you age.

You can improve your ability to think and to create, and you can improve the capacity of your mind as you age; you can improve your ability to concentrate, your ability to solve problems, to plan and to sift and to use new information.

Each individual brain cell (and, remember, there are a million million of them) is constantly trying to make connections with as many other cells as it possibly can.

All the brain cells are independent but they are also interdependent – they want to form as many connections as they can with other cells because it is through the connections they form that they are able to 'communicate'.

If the cells in a baby's brain are not stimulated they will not connect with one another. It is only when cells are encouraged to connect with other cells that the brain really starts to develop.

The difference between a boring, routine, dull, obedient, predictable individual and a lively, inventive, creative, thoughtful individual lies not in the number of brain cells but in the number of connections there are between the brain cells.

Clearly, therefore, intelligence is not so much related to the number of brain cells, or the size of the brain cells, as to the number of connections there are between all the existing brain cells.

And the good news is that by exercising your brain the right way you can increase the number of connections.

If you use the right triggers you can encourage your brain to become more powerful and constantly to increase its potential for calculation, memory and creativity.

Your brain can grow as you age – not only becoming more complex but also becoming more agile and more creative. There is no practical reason why your brain should not improve in efficiency right until the moment that your body expires.

Our brains have a far greater capacity than most of us ever get close to realising. Indeed, each individual brain cell has far greater potential than we ever realise.

If you know how to exercise your brain properly it is possible to reverse any apparent decline in intelligence which may accompany the onset of Alzheimer's disease, or follow a stroke.

Using your mind will help develop surplus brain tissue which will help to compensate for the tissue which has been damaged by Alzheimer's disease, and will help to create new routes around the sort of damage done by a stroke.

Keep your mind active you will enhance your chances of staying healthy and living to celebrate your 100th birthday.

To the extent that it can be improved and kept powerful by regular exercise the brain is not dissimilar to a muscle.

***

A quick look through the history books will confirm that many of the world's most notable geniuses produced their greatest achievements when they were at or beyond what would now be regarded as 'retirement' age.

Michelangelo began work on St Peter's at the age of 63, Leonardo da Vinci was 52 when he started painting the *Mona Lisa*, Brahms didn't write a symphony until he was 43, Verdi wrote two of his greatest operas after the age of 70. German literary giant Johann Goethe finished writing *Faust* at the age of 81.

Painters Henri Matisse and Claude Monet did some of their greatest work in their early 80s. Antonio Stradivari was still making violins at the age of 93.

Writer H.G. Wells was awarded a DSc for a doctoral thesis at the age of 78. American actor George Burns won an Oscar at the age of 80. William Gladstone became British Prime Minister for the fourth time at the age of 82 – and at the same age Winston Churchill published the first part of his four volume work *A History of the English Speaking Peoples*.

You will also find, if you look at the ages at which great men and women died, that professional writers, artists, musicians and others who fully exercised their mental faculties lived – barring accidents – considerably longer than people who worked for large organisations and retired early to play golf or tend to their roses.

How often have you heard someone say: 'What a shame! He worked hard all his life, retired and then died before he could enjoy his retirement!'?

***

If you are over 30 then you have probably got into the habit of assuming that every memory failure is a consequence of old age. This is, of course, a self-fulfilling nonsense. Your assumption that memory falters with age is based purely on the myth that we are all constantly losing brain cells. Having accepted the myth you expect your brain to deteriorate and when you find a sign (such as a temporary incidence of forgetfulness) that suggests a mental weakness you take this as just another piece of evidence supporting the myth.

The fact is, of course, that children and teenagers forget things too. But they don't blame their temporary memory loss, or even regular forgetfulness, on brain decay.

The myth of elderly brain decay is given extra impetus by the fact that a high percentage of individuals over the age of 50 regularly take prescription drugs (such as sleeping tablets) which can cause confusion and forgetfulness. A high percentage of prescription drugs regularly cause mental symptoms, but the link between the individual drugs and the mental symptoms is rarely recognised. Instead of reducing or changing a drug, the medical response is usually to increase the dosage – thereby making things worse.

I hate to think how many patients there are in hospitals, nursing homes, rest homes and back bedrooms who have been diagnosed as suffering from senile dementia but who are, in reality, suffering from nothing more significant than a drug side effect, and who could live happily and fulfilling lives if their doctor stopped their medication. (Drug therapy must, of course, always be stopped by a doctor. Stopping drugs may need special care.)

***

The really exciting news is that your brain can be exercised – and its effectiveness improved – just as easily as your body can be exercised and improved. You can expand the power of your brain through exercise. If you exercise your brain the right way you can preserve and even improve your brain – and your mental powers – even though you are ageing.

The more you use your brain the more you will improve the number of connections. The greater the number of connections there are between individual brain cells the greater the power of your brain will be. Naturally, the greater your brainpower the greater will be your chance of success in your chosen areas of life.

(It is not by chance that many national Olympic squads now spend as much as a third of their training time working on positive thinking, visualisation and mind games. A healthy, creative and positive mind is just as important for success in any field as a healthy body.)

However hard you may find it to exercise your mind – and use your brain properly – you can take comfort from the fact that the more you learn and the more you use your mind the easier learning and thinking creatively will become.

If you think of your brain as a computer then by constantly working it you will expand its memory and capacity. Exercise your mind regularly and you will increase the number of synaptic connections – thus increasing the capability of your brain. A bigger computer will have greater capabilities and will work faster.

Naturally, you have to learn to use the left side of your brain (which handles language, numbers, logic, analysis and lists) with the right side of your brain (which controls colour, imagination, dimension, rhythm and instinct).

***

Here are my 22 tips on exactly how you can improve your mental skills and agility and the power of your brain as you age.

1. Never stop learning.

If you stop learning then your brain will atrophy. The easiest way to improve your brain is to constantly set it new challenges. The more you learn the easier you will find it to learn. The tragedy is that many people over the age of fifty have forgotten how to learn. They have fallen into a groove (or a rut) and are poorly motivated. Your brain needs regular supplies of oxygen, and nutrition but it also needs regular supplies of information. You can supply it with the first two by eating sensibly and taking regular exercise. You can supply the third by making sure that you never stop learning.

2. Look for new challenges

You can help maintain and improve your mental alertness throughout middle age and old age by taking on new experiences and being prepared to accept change in your life. Try to look upon new circumstances as exciting challenges. If you settle down into a comfortable rut then your brain will start to atrophy. If you are for ever looking for fresh challenges and new stimulation you will find that your life will become much richer and infinitely more fun. A life which is without challenge is a life without meaning. The wider and more varied the challenges you take on the greater you will benefit. Winston Churchill's hobbies included brick laying (and building walls) and painting landscapes. The more you challenge your mind the more new brain circuitry you will build.

3. Stay involved in life and with other people

Mental deterioration is most marked among people who stop communicating with others. The more people you meet – and the more interest you take in their lives and their problems – the better your brain will become. A twenty year study of 4,000 people showed that elderly people who take on responsibilities and maintain active social lives end up being able to do far more than people who lead limited and restricted lives. It is perhaps also worth mentioning here that love (both emotional and physical) plays a vital role in maintaining good mental health. Research has shown that we are all healthier when we are loved, cuddled and touched by those whom we ourselves love.

4. Maintain good physical health

If you're going to keep your brain in good condition it is obviously important to preserve your general health. Avoid smoking, take regular physical exercise and eat a healthy diet.

5. Stretch your brain.

Just as you exercise your body so you can exercise your mind by using mind games. Games and puzzles which make you think will also improve your mental powers – and keep you thinking young. It has been shown that mental games – such as chess, backgammon, card games, crossword puzzles and so on – will all help to keep your brain in good shape. The best games require memory, mental discipline, coolness under pressure, insight, an ability to create a strategy, an ability to spot opportunities and assess risks and probabilities.

6. Don't be afraid to be different

Do not allow yourself to be conned into behaving as you think you are expected to behave. Many people in their fifties or sixties or older feel that they have to act with decorum, dress in a certain way and generally behave in a sensible and respectable fashion. They feel that they will shock people if they begin new careers or start new relationships at that age. Why care what other people think? Don't be pushed into acting your age. Act the age you feel.

7. You need a purpose

A clear vision of what you want – and how you are going to get it – will concentrate your mind and vastly improve your brainpower. Constant effort without purpose and direction is inevitably meaningless. Motivate and focus yourself and your energies by giving yourself a purpose and you will add meaning to your life. People who achieve all their ambitions tend to die quite quickly afterwards.

8. Be determined and persistent
Albert Einstein once admitted that: 'Curiosity, obsession and dogged endurance, combined with self-criticism, have brought me my ideas.'

9. Think creatively
Instead of allowing yourself to think only in a linear fashion try thinking laterally and vertically too.

10. Learn to read faster
When you are looking at documents merely in order to sift and sort through information you need to be able to speed read. (You can, of course, read as slowly as you like when reading purely for pleasure). You may find that using a pointer (a finger, a ruler or a pencil) will help you focus directly on the part of the page you are reading. And try to look at two or three words – or even a whole line of type – at once, rather than concentrating on individual letters of words.

11. Listen to music
I have written elsewhere, for example in my book *How to Conquer Pain* (published by the European Medical Journal) about the value of music. There is, however, also evidence to show that listening to certain types of music can be mentally invigorating and may even improve a measurable IQ level. Listening to music by Mozart and Beethoven is particularly recommended.

12. Reject the word 'impossible'
Be regularly on the look out for new challenges. Make a list of the things you've always wanted to do. And start working your way down your list.

13. Develop your sense of humour
Few skills will help you deal with life – and stay positive, optimistic and active – more effectively than a well developed sense of humour.

14. Remain physically active
You may not be able to run a mile but that doesn't mean that you can't walk a mile. Remain as physically active as you possibly can.

15. Alcohol can be a boon
Research has shown that elderly male drinkers (who drink sensibly and limit their consumption of alcohol to no more than one or two modest drinks a day) score better in intelligence tests than non-drinkers. But remember the word 'sensible'. Drinking too much can wreck your brain as rapidly as any other drug. And many, such as those with addictive personalities or liver disease, should not drink alcohol at all.

16. Learn to commit yourself – and to begin!
You'll never finish if you don't start. Prevarication is the commonest cause of failure. If you have always wanted to write a novel then start writing one. It doesn't matter if you have to throw away the first fifty pages – just beginning will open up your mind to the possibility of success.

17. Live with an animal
I have for decades argued that living with animals helps keep people healthy, and a great deal of research has been done to support this claim. Researchers examined 5,741 people and found that people who lived with 'pet' animals had significantly lower blood pressure and lower levels of cholesterol – and were less stressed mentally. Research in nursing homes has often shown that patients who are allowed to have pets are much healthier than other patients. (And yet there are still some doctors and administrators who object to patients in such homes keeping pets). The value of a pet has been underestimated by those who do not realise that a pet can be just as much a friend and a companion as another human being.

18. Be prepared to take naps
Leonardo da Vinci took 15-minute naps every four hours or so. There is a good deal of sense in following his example. You are likely to awake refreshed and able to think better and more clearly.

19. Drink plenty of fresh water
Water will help clear out toxins. But limit your consumption of caffeine-rich drinks such as coffee and tea.

20. Get into the habit of making lists
Help your mind and stimulate your memory by using lists and making notes. Use coloured pens and always keep a pen and notebook handy so that you can scrawl memos to yourself.

21. Lose any excess weight
The brains of people who are overweight get less oxygen when they are

asleep. Obese people who lose weight may reverse the damage which has been done and become intellectually brighter.

22. Concentrate more

As your brain gets older so your ability to remember things that you have looked at briefly will get worse. When you were young you could probably look at a list of words and remember quite a lot of them. You may not be able to do that as easily when you're older. You may need to concentrate more. To remember where you parked the car you will need to make a conscious effort. Look at your car and its surroundings to imprint the view on your memory. Pretend that you are taking a photograph of it – blink your eyelids as though your eyes were cameras – and you'll remember it better.

Normally we remember around 20% of what we read. But if you really concentrate you can remember up to 70%. After reading something that you want to remember spend 60 seconds thinking about it. Make a mental comment to yourself about what you have read. Rephrase it in your mind. You will find that if you do this your memory will improve considerably.

As we get older we all do things without really thinking about them. We put ourselves onto 'automatic pilot' and fall into a routine. Concentrate really hard and spot the things you do without thinking. And then ask yourself whether or not you could do things better if you thought about them more.

Try to understand things that you have to remember. You will find things easier to remember if you understand them. And try to remember key facts and key words which will help bring into your mind whole sequences of thoughts and facts.

If you want to remember important things try clearing your brain of trivial information. Use notebooks and diaries to record trivial material. Albert Einstein once said: 'Why should I waste brain space remembering my own telephone number? I can look it up if I want to know what it is.'

When you are talking about something you know that you will want to remember try to concentrate hard on everything around you. Concentrate on the people you are with and the place you are in. Try to be aware of smells, sights and sounds. The more information you record the easier you will find it to remember the event. If you want to remember something that you have seen or read try closing your eyes immediately afterwards. This keeps the 'image' on your retina for a little longer – and will make the image easier to recall in the future.

When you are trying to remember something do your best to recreate the conditions under which you learnt it. Football teams do best when playing at home (even if there isn't a crowd of home supporters) because they find it easier to remember what they've learned while training. Students do better in examinations if they take their tests in the room where they did their learning. So, if you are trying to remember the name of someone you met at a party then try to remember where you were, what you were doing, what you were wearing, what other people were wearing and what you said to the people you met. Things that you learn are bound together in your mind in time and place. If you can recreate the conditions in which you learned something then your ability to recall the facts will increase dramatically. If you are struggling to remember something work your way through the alphabet. The first letter of a name or place can often 'trigger' a lost memory.

To make it easier to remember names try to make up pictures in your mind. For example, to remember the name 'Coleman' think of a man carrying a bag of coal. If you are trying to remember a name like 'Vernon' which doesn't lend itself to a picture then visualise an imaginary blackboard in your mind and then write the name onto your blackboard. When you want to recall the name simply recreate your blackboard.

Chapter Fourteen

Use Anti-oxidants To Overcome The Evil Of Free Radicals

Free radicals contribute to heart disease, stroke and dementia. Arthritis, various types of cancer and brain problems such as Parkinson's disease are also all believed to be caused by free radicals. Even cataracts are believed to be caused by damage caused by free radicals.

And yet despite the fact that there is excellent research showing that anti-oxidants such as vitamin E and selenium can help prevent these free radical induced problems, most doctors still fail to tell their patients about anti-oxidants.

One important study showed that patients who took vitamin E every day were less likely to die, need to be institutionalised, develop Alzheimer's disease or lose the ability to look after their own daily needs. Another survey showed that the progress of coronary artery disease was slower in men who took vitamin E every day than in men who didn't take such a supplement. Another survey showed that men who consumed decent amounts of dietary vitamin E had half the risk of coronary artery disease of men who consumed very low amounts of the vitamin. And one study found that women who took vitamin E for two years had half the coronary artery disease risk of women not taking the vitamin.

Taking selenium daily seems to help too. A study in the Netherlands showed that low selenium levels are associated with an increased heart attack risk. A study in the *Journal of the American Medical Association* showed that when patients who had suffered from skin cancer were given daily selenium they were less likely to die from cancer than patients who were not given selenium. When those conducting this study also found that the individuals who received selenium had two thirds the risk of developing any additional form of cancer and half the risk of dying from cancer, they stopped the study in its sixth year so that the people in the comparison group could be given the chance to take selenium. It is remarkable that cancer patients who take selenium are 50% less likely to die of their cancer than those who don't. Don't be tempted to take too much selenium. It can build up to toxic levels.

Vitamin C is a crucial part of any healthy diet. I don't believe that taking vitamin C will automatically stop you getting colds. But if you don't eat a daily diet which is rich in fruits and vegetables then it may be wise to take a daily supplement. Vitamin A is useful as an anti-oxidant but probably not as useful as a cancer fighter as C and E. Don't take too much and take it as beta carotene. Too much vitamin A can be dangerous (and can do far more harm than good) but your body won't convert beta carotene into vitamin A unless it needs it. Smokers shouldn't take vitamin A since vitamin A − even when taken in the safer beta carotene form − is toxic when combined with cigarette smoke.

Grape seed contains pyrocyanidines, known as potent anti-oxidants. Grape seed extract seems safe as well as useful.

While on the subject of vitamins it is worth mentioning that vegans, who may get their B12 only from fortified foods may need to take a supplement of B12.

For years I opposed the use of vitamin and mineral supplements. I've changed my mind. I think they are now vital. I recommend taking a supplement which contains vitamin C, vitamin E, selenium and grape seed extract. Do use supplements wisely. Don't indiscriminately take vitamin or mineral supplements. You can do yourself more harm than good by taking the wrong vitamins or, even, the right vitamins in the wrong dosage.

Chapter Fifteen

Could Your Illness Be Caused By An Allergy?

Allergies are a rapidly growing problem. More people than ever now suffer from disorders traditionally recognised as being allergy-induced – disorders such as asthma, eczema and hay fever. During the 1980s the number of people seeking medical advice for asthma and hay fever doubled. Today one in seven school children carries an inhaler for asthma. (Although, as I have explained elsewhere, this may be partly because doctors now diagnose these problems more readily.)

But there is now a growing amount of evidence to show that a far greater variety of symptoms – and diseases – may be caused by an allergy response. And many experts now recognise that this is due to the fact that we are surrounded by a bigger variety of chemicals and other environmental contaminants than were our ancestors. Some of these chemicals are in the air we breathe and the water we drink and a great many are in the food we eat.

(The field of medicine that used to be described as including allergy problems is now sometimes described as environmental medicine and sometimes as clinical ecology. This is a rapidly developing area of health care but far more research needs to be done before we understand all the links between allergens and symptoms.)

Symptoms and disorders now recognised as possibly being allergy disorders include: arthritis, irritable bowel syndrome, migraine, mood swings, muscle pains and a wide variety of other mental and physical disorders.

Despite the fact that it is now widely recognised that allergy problems are on the rise, that allergy symptoms are often caused by chemical contaminants and that the number of chemical contaminants in our environment is constantly growing there is much ignorance and scepticism among doctors and other health care professionals, and many practitioners are still quicker to reach for their prescription pads than they are to look for a possible allergy link when they find themselves faced with a patient suffering from a chronic and apparently intractable health problem.

The result can be disastrous not only because many patients suffer from long term health problems which may last for years, or even decades, and ruin their lives but also because the drugs which are prescribed as remedies may themselves turn out to create additional allergy problems.

There obviously isn't room here to detail every possible allergen and every disorder which can be caused by an allergic response.

But in a way that really doesn't matter because allergy problems are often unique to individual patients and a textbook that was as thick as twelve telephone directories could not include all the possible combinations of allergens and symptoms. A fully comprehensive list of known allergens would have to include just about every substance known to man.

What I do intend to do – and what I think you will find far more useful – is to give you information which might help you to decide whether or not a specific symptom (or set of symptoms) might be caused by an allergy response.

However, before I go any further I must include a couple of warnings.

First (and most important) it is extremely important that you do not assume that undiagnosed symptoms are caused by an allergic problem. Symptoms which can be allergy related (such as wheezing or headaches) may also be caused by other underlying disorders – some of which may be serious and potentially life threatening.

Second, it is also important to remember that some of the symptoms which are often thought of as being linked to an allergy of some kind may be a perfectly normal (and healthy) response to a threat from outside the body. So, for example, a sneeze may be a sign of a developing allergy response but it may also be the body's way of protecting itself. Similarly, watering eyes may be a sign of an allergy problem but they may be the body's attempt to wash a foreign body of some kind out of the eye. When such symptoms are brought into action as part of the body's own protective mechanism it may be important to leave them alone. Interfering with, or attempting to suppress, the body's self-healing mechanisms may create new problems. (I have dealt with the body's self-healing and self-protecting powers in my book *Bodypower* which is published by the European Medical Journal.)

***

When your body detects an allergen – which it regards as a threat – it releases its own internal chemicals in order to protect itself. These chemicals may result in the contraction or spasm of muscles, an increase in the production of mucus and the dilatation of small blood vessels. As a result of those changes the following symptoms may develop:

- Fatigue and exhaustion
- Anxiety
- Depression
- Hyperactivity
- Food craving or addiction
- Epilepsy
- Headache
- Migraine
- Itchy eyes
- Runny nose
- Blocked nose
- Sneezing
- Blocked sinuses
- Breathing through the nose
- Inflamed sinuses
- Ear infections
- Wheezing
- Tight chest
- Hoarseness
- Persistent coughing
- Indigestion
- Diarrhoea
- Vomiting
- Nausea
- Colitis
- Intestinal spasm
- Wind
- Constipation
- Mouth ulcers
- Red skin
- Dry, scaly skin
- Itchy skin
- Nettle rash
- Swollen tissues/water retention
- Joint pains
- Muscle pains
- Menstrual symptoms

If you are suffering from an allergy disorder then you could be suffering from one, two, more or conceivably all of the above symptoms. But, obviously, not all these symptoms are always caused by allergies. The symptom pattern is the key to diagnosing an allergy problem.

So how do you tell whether or not your particular symptoms could be allergy related? Obviously, there are some tests that doctors can organise. But I believe that too much emphasis and reliance is sometimes put on laboratory tests – and too little on using detective work to try and decide whether or not a particular set of symptoms are or could be allergy related. Laboratory tests are often complicated, sometimes painful, frequently unreliable, occasionally dangerous and invariably expensive. Using detective work to help you decide whether a certain set of symptoms could be allergy related – and if so what to – should be simple, painless, reliable, safe and inexpensive.

It is worth remembering that although any allergen may produce virtually any symptom, or set of symptoms, it does seem that allergens which are inhaled are most likely to produce breathing and nasal symptoms, that intestinal problems are more likely to be caused by allergens which are swallowed and that skin symptoms are often caused by substances with which the skin has been in contact. You must also remember that allergy symptoms can often be delayed. It is common for symptoms to occur six hours after contact but there may be a delay of a day or more. This means that it is quite likely that your allergy symptoms will only develop quite late at night (or early the following morning) after encountering an allergen.

I've put together a list of some fairly basic rules that should help you decide. And to make the list easier to use I've put the rules into question form.

1. Are your symptoms seasonal – i.e. do they occur only at certain times of the year? When symptoms follow this pattern it is a clear indication that there is a good chance that you are allergic to some type of pollen or mould spore.

2. Did something in your life change at the same time as your symptoms started? Did you change your job? Acquire a new pet? Start to use a new type of washing powder? Buy a new carpet or piece of clothing? Start taking a drug? Eat something that you hadn't eaten before?

3. Do your symptoms often or always start or get worse after you've eaten a particular type of food, visited a particular place or worn certain clothes? Remember that there may be a delay of some hours between the contact with the allergen and the development of symptoms.

4. Are your symptoms constant? If there is very little variation in your symptoms from hour to hour or day to day and you have an allergy problem then the chances are that the cause of your problem will be

something you eat, drink or wear every day – or some chemical with which you are in contact on a daily basis. It is, however, also possible that you may be responding to several (or many) different allergens.

5. Do your symptoms disappear or improve at the weekends or when you go away on holiday? If this is the pattern that your symptoms follow then the chances are high that you are allergic to something with which you come into contact at work.

If, after studying these questions, you still can't find a link then try keeping a 'symptoms diary'. Write down details of when your symptoms develop (or are at their worst), what time of day it is and what you are doing at the time.

***

There aren't many substances which can't cause allergy symptoms – or which haven't caused allergy symptoms in someone at some time, although substances which are extremely inert (such as stone, marble, cork and glass) are unlikely to cause problems unless they have been treated with chemicals (such as paints and varnishes) which are likely to cause problems.

It is worth remembering that stress, extreme heat, extreme cold, too much exercise, an infection and an unusually high or unusually low blood sugar level, may all increase the body's susceptibility to allergens. Some women find that they get allergy symptoms only when they are menstruating or ovulating. It is also possible for an exposure to one powerful allergen to trigger a reaction to other allergens which might, under normal circumstances, have failed to produce much, if anything, in the way of symptoms. Finally, it may also be useful to know that when products which can cause symptoms have been allowed to air they may cause fewer problems than they did when they were new.

Here is a list of some common allergens.

1. Tobacco smoke
Extremely common – and often a cause of severe symptoms.

2. Vehicle exhaust fumes and industrial smokes

3. Gas and paraffin fumes

4. Cleaning products (e.g. bleach, detergent)
It is not uncommon for allergy problems to develop as a result of wearing clothes which have been washed in powerful detergents. Also remember that you may be allergic to cleaning products used in public buildings (if a public building is visited regularly symptoms may be virtually permanent).

5. Cosmetics and toiletries
Remember that it is possible to acquire an allergy to someone else's perfume. Regular contact may produce regular symptoms whereas occasional or isolated contact (for example sitting next to someone on a train) may cause occasional or isolated symptoms.

6. Drinking water
Chlorine and other chemicals which have been deliberately put into the water may be mixed with contaminants.

7. Adhesives, solvents and paints
Chemicals used in the manufacture of magazines and newspapers and in some office equipment may cause problems. The fumes given off within a newly painted room are particularly likely to cause trouble.

8. Bedding and clothing
Chemicals in synthetic materials may cause symptoms as may dyes and washing powders.

9. Furniture, flooring and fabrics
Chemicals used in the manufacture of chairs, carpets, curtains and other household items may cause symptoms. You should also note that the plastics and foams used in the manufacture of modern motor cars may cause symptoms. More fumes are produced by the chemical products in new cars, and hot days seem to make matters even worse. The plastics used in the manufacture of television sets and computers can also cause problems.

10. Garden products
Pesticides, insecticides, fungicides and other chemicals can all cause problems.

11. Food
Pesticide residues and deliberately added chemical additives (included as preservatives, colourings, flavourings etc.) can all cause problems. Allergy symptoms caused by foods can be more or less permanent or intermittent. Sometimes they may develop only when a food is eaten in large quantities. It is not unknown for patients who have an allergy to a food which they eat regularly to suffer from constant, troubling, disabling and even life ruining symptoms – aching muscles, headaches, indigestion and inescapable tiredness and exhaustion are common possibilities. Not eating a food which causes problems can sometimes, after a period of weeks or months, result in the allergy disappearing. Alternatively, new and quite different symptoms may

develop. It is also possible for withdrawal symptoms (and these may include: aching muscles, sleep disturbance, tiredness, irritability, nausea, sweating, restlessness, palpitations, skin rash) to develop when a food that has been eaten regularly doesn't appear in the diet.

12. Drugs
Drugs bought over the counter and prescription drugs can both cause problems.

Two Practical Tips For Avoiding Allergies
Please note that if you suffer from severe asthma which you know can be triggered by new products, or you have a had a severe allergy reaction before, then you should take great care before testing any new product.

1. Gently sniff products before you buy them. If you don't like a smell or it makes you feel dizzy or nauseous (or produces other symptoms) then you should probably not buy it. It is worth remembering that if you find a smell particularly attractive then that product may cause problems.
2. If you are about to use a new perfume or some other substance then test the product by dabbing a small amount onto your forearm. Wait 48 hours. If the area of skin reddens, becomes swollen or itchy or shows any other signs of having reacted to the substance then you should obviously not use it.

Chapter Sixteen

Don't Allow Yourself To Be Deceived By Food Company Trickery

There are 76 million cases of food related infectious illnesses in the US every year – with around 5,000 deaths. Figures for other countries are similarly alarming. These figures are probably on the low side. Many people who have short lived illnesses do not bother to report them to anyone. In addition illnesses caused by drinking contaminated water do not count for these figures since water is not regarded as a food. If water borne contamination (and other forms of contamination) were added the total number of incidents of food related infectious illness would exceed 200,000,000 cases a year in the US alone.

Many of these problems are caused by the contamination of food with bacteria, viruses and other organisms. Since human and animal waste is widely used in animal feed this is hardly surprising. (The disgusting practice of feeding faeces to animals is widespread.)

Attempts to control the dramatically increasing problem of food related illness have been futile. Governments everywhere are nervous about upsetting the powerful food industry and even more nervous about upsetting farmers.

Of course, food which is contaminated with infective organisms isn't the only reason why people are falling ill these days. If cases of cancer, heart disease and other diseases caused by diet were added, the numbers involved would be much more dramatic. There is absolutely no doubt that at least a third of all cancers are caused by food. And there are strong links between specific foods and most other major killers too.

In an attempt to stay healthy most of us want to eat nutritious, healthy food that tastes good and does us good. We want to be able to pay a fair price for food that contains natural ingredients and, ideally, no chemical residues. If the food we are buying contains additives we would like to know what they are.

In order to do our best to eat healthily we naturally put a lot of faith in the labels used to describe the food we eat.

Our faith is misplaced.

Encouraged and supported by the government, food companies lie, lie and lie again. Ordinary, everyday words such as 'fresh', 'natural', 'wholesome' and 'nutritious' are virtually meaningless. If the American government has its way the word 'organic' will soon be entirely meaningless too.

We all put our faith in labels – and our trust in the people who sell us food. But our faith and our trust are misplaced. Food companies are aware of our desire for genuinely good food and so they employ clever advertising and marketing 'spin doctors' to help disguise the way that the food they sell us is adulterated by behind-the-scene chemists. The whole food industry has become rather reminiscent of something out of a story by Lewis Carroll.

Here are some of the ways food companies defraud us:

• **Spring water**
The phrase can be used to describe water that has been taken out of a tap.

• **Meat**
The word 'meat' can be used to describe anything that comes from an animal – from the tip of its nose to the tip of its tail. Scraps of meat blasted off the bones are counted, as are bits of faeces clinging to tissues.

• **Farmfresh and Farmhouse**
Utterly meaningless words. The foods described in this way can be produced in factories from animals or birds (such as hens) kept in battery cages.

• **Fresh**
This means whatever the food company wants it to mean.

• **GM Free**
If you think that a 'GM Free' label means that food doesn't contain genetically modified food you would be wrong. (Incidentally, I prefer the phrase genetically engineered.) The rules mean that food can contain a small quantity of genetically modified food and yet be described as not containing genetically modified food. Since the whole point with genetically engineered food is that a small amount may induce cancer this is dangerous and absurd.

• Steak

This implies that the item is a solid piece of flesh. But this isn't necessarily so. 'Steaks' can be built up using scraps and flakes of flesh.

• Low fat

This doesn't mean anything since there are no legal rules defining what 'low fat' means.

• Lean

This doesn't mean anything either. Nor does Extra Lean. (Nor, for that matter, Extra Extra Lean.) A product described as 'lean' may sound as though it contains little fat but it can be just as fatty as any other product.

• Flavour

Don't make the mistake of assuming that the phrase 'banana flavour' implies that the food you are buying has anything to do with bananas. The flavour may be made in a laboratory from chemicals.

• Free range

This doesn't mean that the hens (or other creatures) range free. It means that a vast number of creatures share limited access to a very limited outdoor space. Free range chickens are merely chickens who are technically allowed to stretch their legs. Most are fed on mass produced pellets and never see a hay barn or a blade of grass. Chemicals may be added to the feed in order to try to improve the appearance of the yolks – and in order to keep the hens alive in their unnatural 'free range' conditions. (If you and ten thousand other people lived in one room with a door into a carpet sized garden would you describe yourself as 'free range'?)

• Brown bread

Sounds wholesome but it can be white bread which has been dyed.

• Natural

This word doesn't mean anything when applied to food.

• Smoked

If you think your smoked bacon has been smoked you are probably being naive. Your bacon may well have been pumped up with an artificial smoke flavour liquid.

• Country Fresh Eggs

The hens are probably kept in a battery but the battery may be in the country. The word 'fresh' means whatever the food company wants it to mean.

• Nutritious
This doesn't mean anything at all.

How do food companies get away with all this deceit?
Largely, I'm afraid, because most people don't bother to complain.
What can you do about it?
Become ever more vigilant when buying food.

Chapter Seventeen

Learn To Listen To Your Body's Secret Calls For Help

A friend recently asked me if I could recommend a good back specialist. He told me that he was suffering a lot with back pain and that his family doctor had recommended a hospital appointment.

I didn't know of a back specialist in the area where he lives but, hoping that I might be able to help in some other way, I asked him to tell me a little more about the back trouble he was getting. To get the ball rolling I asked him if he could remember when the back pain had started – and if he could think of anything which made it worse.

It quickly turned out that the back pain had started after my friend had bought a new car – and that the pain was always at its worst when he had been driving in it for a long time. Rather surprisingly, neither my friend nor his doctor had stopped to think that the backache might have a specific cause. Until my question had made him think about it, he hadn't thought about the link between his new pain and his new car.

When I suggested that treating the car might be easier, quicker, cheaper and certainly more effective in the long run than trying to treat his back, my friend was surprised but delighted. He bought himself a back rest and completely got rid of his back problem within days.

It is surprising how often we ignore our bodies when they try to tell us something important. In my friend's case the backache was simply a message from his body complaining about the uncomfortable car. In a surprising number of illnesses it is possible to find that a new symptom is a sign that your body is calling for help.

***

145

Sadly, doctors take very little interest in helping their patients stay healthy. Most of the doctors I've met have been positively hostile towards all aspects of preventive medicine. I find this surprising – and worrying – since it clearly makes more sense to put a little bit of effort into helping to keep someone healthy than to have to spend a large amount of money and time trying to make someone well again.

The problem, however, is that doctors are trained to diagnose and to treat illnesses. The whole emphasis of their training is directed towards the illness rather than the patient. Doctors are not taught how to keep their patients healthy. They receive very little training in psychology and hardly any training at all in nutrition (despite the fact that there is now an enormous amount of evidence to show that stress and the food we eat are probably the two major forces in the development of disease).

Every day of a medical student's training is geared towards diagnosing the disease responsible for a patient's symptoms and then offering one of two main types of treatment: treatment with drugs or surgery. Other therapies offered by doctors, such as radiotherapy, are the only variations on this basic theme.

Doctors are taught to take no interest in patients who do not have any symptoms. The pharmaceutical industry exists to make money from people who are sick. Drug companies aren't interested in preventing disease (either retail or wholesale) and so doctors aren't interested either.

Turn up at your doctor's office and ask him to help you stop smoking or lose weight and you will probably be dismissed within a minute. You will probably be clutching a prescription for an expensive drug company product which, it is claimed, will help you conquer your problem. You may, if you are lucky, also be given a dull and pretty unhelpful leaflet.

Medical students are not taught how to show their patients how to improve their health while receiving orthodox treatment. And they are not taught how to show their patients how to stay healthy when they have been treated.

Anyone who has studied the wider aspects of medicine will readily confirm that it makes clear sense that if you want your body to perform its functions well you should give it the best possible fuel supply. Doctors either don't know this or else they ignore it. Spend time in hospital and you may find yourself expected to defeat your illness on a diet of over-cooked junk food.

Common, serious diseases such as heart disease, high blood pressure and osteoporosis can, in the vast majority of cases, be prevented or treated simply, easily, cheaply and effectively. For most sufferers of these disorders pharmaceutical company products are an expensive and toxic irrelevance.

Remember that your biggest ally in your aim to stay healthy is your body. Your body's sole aim is to protect and preserve itself. The Cartesian view of the body as a machine is woefully inadequate (and yet it is still regarded as a fundamental truth by most medical researchers and members of the medical establishment) for how many machines can avoid danger and repair themselves?

Despite the obvious truth of all this most people still ignore their bodies (and refuse to listen when their bodies are talking to them) and prefer to put their faith in the hands of doctors − a group of former professionals whose education has for decades been under the control of an industry.

***

Many, many years ago I used to provide regular medical advice for viewers of a British breakfast television station. I remember that one morning I told viewers that in order to spot early signs of illness they should learn to 'listen to their bodies'. Two days later I received a letter from a woman viewer who told me off for offering advice she couldn't take. She said that she couldn't listen to her body because she was deaf.

That was not, of course, quite what I meant. Being able to listen to your body requires a general state of awareness and is one of the fundamental building stones upon which continuing good health is based.

Instead of listening to our bodies, and taking note of those secret calls for help, we tend to regard all symptoms as unwelcome.

And yet if you do learn to listen to your body it is often possible to spot physical and mental symptoms at a very early stage and to take action to avoid more lasting damage. Over the years I have distilled and refined my thoughts on this topic. (See my book *Bodypower* for a fuller description of my thoughts on the body's self healing powers.)

In order to provide a practical illustration of precisely what I mean here are just two examples of common cries for help which are frequently either ignored or simply smothered with powerful medication without any attention being paid to the possibility that there may be an underlying cause which can be tackled. Smothering symptoms with a drug may produce temporary relief but it isn't likely to produce any lasting cure, and the chances are that the underlying problem, whatever it is, will simply continue to get worse.

Example 1: Sleeplessness

If you can't get to sleep at night there is usually a reason. Taking sleeping tablets may help you get to sleep (for a while) but the reason will still be there. The underlying problem which is keeping you awake may lie within your body (pain or breathlessness for example); within your mind (anxiety about a domestic or occupational problem for example) or outside both your body and your mind (noisy plumbing, noisy neighbours or a freezing cold bedroom).

Example 2: Indigestion

If five people sit down to dinner there is a good chance that by the time the meal is over one of them will have indigestion. Most people treat indigestion as a mild annoyance – most commonly swallowing antacid medicine or tablets to banish the pain. If the indigestion occurs very rarely (once a year) then this isn't too daft. But if the indigestion occurs commonly then this is a pretty silly thing to do. Unless something is done about the cause of the problem then the chances are high that the trouble will simply recur – and may lead to more serious problems developing. Indigestion may be a warning sign that the individual concerned is exposed to too much stress, is eating the wrong foods, eating too quickly or overusing tobacco or alcohol. It is a major indictment of the modern medical profession that nine out of ten doctors will treat indigestion, gastritis or peptic ulceration as a 'disease' to be treated rather than as a sign that a lifestyle change is called for.

If you're going to deal with the underlying cause of an illness (rather than merely tackle the superficial symptom or symptoms) then you need to become something of a medical detective.

Whenever there is something wrong with you (physically or mentally) ask yourself what your body might be trying to tell you.

I think that the phrase I used on TV all those years ago still sums up this approach: learn to listen to your body. Your body knows far more than you think it does – and it has a great deal to tell you.

Chapter Eighteen

Medical Screening Programmes Do More Harm Than Good

It is well over a decade since I first warned about the futility of breast screening programmes (very shortly after these expensive and highly profitable programmes had been introduced).

Since 1988 I have been convinced that the potential health hazards which may be associated with mammograms could outweigh the advantages. This conviction was not based on any inside knowledge. It always seemed to me pretty obvious that repeatedly subjecting breast tissue (which is known to be prone to cancer) to X-rays (which is known to cause cancer) could be hazardous. This seems to me to be a fairly obvious concern. But it is one which the medical establishment has regularly dismissed as not even worth consideration. (Relatively recent research has shown that one woman in every 1,000 screened will develop breast cancer in the two years following the X-ray.)

It seems to me that the risks associated with mammograms should have been properly assessed before mass mammography was introduced.

(I do, however, recommend that women learn to examine their own breasts regularly for this is, I believe, an excellent way to ensure that lumps are spotted early.)

***

Fear about the danger of mammography isn't my only concern about medical screening programmes. Medical screening programmes can produce two types of error: false negatives and false positives.

A false negative occurs when the screening programme misses a genuine cancer. For example, one in four breast cancers go undetected by mammography.

149

And a false positive occurs when the screening programme picks up what appears to be a cancer in a healthy breast.

(Both types of error are acknowledged problems in all screening programmes.)

When there is a false negative result the main danger is obviously that a condition requiring treatment will be missed. But there is also a risk that the woman concerned may ignore – or dismiss – a lump which she feels in the bath, when dressing or when examining her own breasts because she has been given an official 'all clear'.

False positives can lead to unnecessary tests, surgery, mutilation and potentially lethal chemotherapy.

One major survey (involving 600,000 women aged between 50 and 60) suggested that official breast screening may not produce any significant reduction in fatalities.

This survey showed that 100,000 of the 600,000 women had been falsely diagnosed as having cancer. Of these 16,000 had undergone biopsy and more than 400 had had surgery – including mastectomy. In addition, of course, all those 100,000 women (and their partners) will have been exposed to tremendous anxiety and stress – and many immune systems will have been damaged as a result (ironically, increasing the likelihood of cancer developing).

The medical establishment's response to this new evidence was not to call for official breast screening programmes to be stopped, or even to be reassessed, but to call for the breast screening programmes to be extended to include more women – and more screening. (This is the usual response when the truth tends to threaten a profitable medical enterprise.)

***

For decades now just about every attempt to show that medical screening programmes save lives has proved that they are a waste of time, energy and money. Surveys have proved that because of the risk of false positives medical screening programmes do more harm than good.

Medical screening programmes go back a long way. The first recorded screening took place at a public brothel in Avignon in 1347 when a local Abbess and a surgeon examined all the working women every Saturday to see whether or not they were fit to carry on serving the local population.

Modern screening really started in 1917 in the US when large corporations thought it might be a good idea to have their employees examined regularly. When half of four million American men called up for military service during the first World War proved to be unfit for military service insurance companies started screening the general population.

Since then the medical screening business has grown virtually unchecked – despite the fact that since the 1970s there has been ample evidence to show that medical screening programmes are not just a waste of time and money but can also be a serious health hazard.

Back in 1979, the World Health Organization published a report which showed that people who were subjected to regular medical screenings needed to go to hospital more often but were not as healthy as people who did not undergo regular medical screenings. The conclusion was that health screening is expensive and ineffective.

In the same year (1979) the results of a Canadian Task Force report on Periodic Health Examination came to the conclusion that annual medical check-ups should be abandoned since they are both inefficient and potentially harmful.

**

Those who have studied general health screening programmes with an open mind have come to the conclusion that they are harmful for four reasons.

First, when people are taught to put their faith in medical check-ups they tend to abandon responsibility for their own health and enjoy a false sense of security. Patients forget that a medical check-up is no more a sign of long term health than an encouraging bank statement is a sign of permanent financial security. A patient who is given a clean bill of health is likely to ignore strange symptoms which develop a week or two later. And there is a danger that he (or she) may feel that it is unnecessary to eat wisely or to take regular exercise.

Second, screening examinations may frighten people. They can result in cancer phobias, neuroses and depression. And they can result in so much stress that the immune system is damaged – leading to a greater susceptibility to disease.

Third, the procedures involved in screening programmes may do physical harm. There are, for example, some doctors who perform coronary angiographs as part of their check-up procedures. As many as two patients per 100 may die during this procedure.

Fourth, when a screening examination results in a false positive the patient may be given a treatment which may damage his or her health. The report on breast screening which I quoted above showed that out of 600,000 women screened there had been 100,000 false positives.

**

Why, when the evidence shows so clearly that medical screening is a waste of time, does the medical establishment remain so enthusiastic?

Every independent survey I have found has concluded that screening (whether general or specific) is costly and useless. The only people who benefit from screening programmes are doctors – and other parts of the health industry. Screening programmes are extremely profitable.

I find it difficult to avoid the conclusion that the medical profession (and the wider medical industry) remain enthusiastic about screening – despite the evidence – simply because medical screening is a hugely profitable business.

***

The best way to spot health problems early is to learn to listen to your own body.

Be aware of how your body feels – and reacts – when it is healthy and you will be much more likely to be aware when things go wrong.

You should seek advice from a properly trained and qualified health care professional whom you trust if:

1. You have any unexplained pain which recurs or which is present for more than five days (obviously, severe, uncontrollable pain needs to be investigated without delay).
2. You have any unexplained bleeding – from anywhere.
3. You need to take any home medicine regularly or for five days or more.
4. You notice any persistent change in your body (e.g. a loss or gain in weight, a paralysis of any kind, or the development of any lump or swelling).
5. Any existing lump, wart or other skin blemish changes size or colour, or bleeds.
6. You notice new symptoms when you have already received medical treatment.
7. There are mental symptoms present such as confusion, paranoia, disorientation or severe depression.

Chapter Nineteen

When Tests And Investigations Need To Be Ignored

It has always seemed to me that one of the fundamental principles by which any doctor should practise medicine is that it is the patient, not the laboratory test, which should be treated. It is sad that this is often not the case these days.

Tests and investigations can, of course, be helpful. But in my view (and I recognise that this is probably not a widely held view among doctors) it is an abdication of professional responsibility to allow test results to take priority over the patient's symptoms. Perhaps more doctors should have faith in their instincts and judgements.

***

The first thing that everyone (patients and doctors) should remember is that test results can be wrong.

This may sound rather blasphemous. We are all encouraged to believe that when a machine spews out a piece of paper containing lists of figures the result must be accurate. When results come back from the laboratory they are regarded with the sort of reverence once accorded to messages on tablets of stone.

But the fact is that most laboratory tests are only 95% accurate.

If a test to detect a disease, whose prevalence is one in 1,000, has a false positive rate of 5%, there will be 51 positive results if 1,000 people are tested. Of those 51 patients with positive results just one will actually have the disease concerned. The other 50 will appear to have the disease but will, in reality, be healthy. (When considering this remarkable figure you should remember that the prevalence rate for many diseases is much less than 1 in 1,000. A false positive rate of 5% for a disease which affects 1 in 1,000,000 people will mean that 50,001 people have positive results but only one of them actually has the disease concerned.)

Furthermore, that 95% accuracy rate which I have quoted is only reliable when all the equipment in the laboratory is working absolutely perfectly – this is something that usually happens about once a week. As a general rule 90% accuracy is more likely.

All this assumes that all the technicians involved do their jobs perfectly and never make mistakes. As has been shown many times in recent years human error can be extremely significant – and can cause catastrophic results, much illness and many deaths.

And, of course, most patients have more than one test done. If a patient has twenty laboratory tests done (not at all unusual) then there is a good chance that even if the patient is perfectly healthy the tests will show at least one abnormality.

When doctors spot an abnormality on a test report they immediately think of disease and then they think of treatment. There is a tendency to forget or ignore the condition of the patient.

It is easy to see from all this that every patient going into hospital will have a good chance of being treated for a disease he or she hasn't got.

Even when no treatment is given there is a good chance that when a false diagnosis is made a patient's life may be changed. One recent study showed that out of 93 children who had been diagnosed as having heart disease – and who had lived their lives as 'heart patients' – only 17 really had heart disease.

When the first blood test for syphilis was introduced doctors accepted it as accurate. It wasn't until several decades later that doctors found that 50% of all patients whose blood test had shown them to have syphilis didn't have syphilis at all. The lives of many of those patients must have been ruined quite unnecessarily.

***

Of course, if there is a chance that a laboratory error may mean that a normal sample results in a 'false positive' there must also be a chance that a laboratory error may mean that an abnormal sample results in a 'false negative' reading.

A 'false negative' reading means that many patients who have symptoms and signs of an underlying illness will be falsely reassured that there is nothing wrong with them.

The doctor (or the patient) may make a diagnosis and then, when the laboratory results come back, assume that the diagnosis must be wrong.

My guess (and this is only a guess because I am not aware of any scientific research on this subject) is that when faced with a patient with clear cut symptoms strongly indicating an underlying problem, and a set of 'normal' laboratory results, the vast majority of doctors will allow themselves to be influenced more by the laboratory results than by the patient's condition and their own clinical experience.

***

Next, we should consider the fact that, much as the technicians might dislike and dispute this, I do not believe that everyone fits neatly into the range of 'normal values'.

We are all different (for which we should thank God, though if the genetic engineers get their own way and cloning becomes commonplace this will no longer be true) and the whole concept of 'normal values' is an entirely artificial one. It should be used only as a guideline, rather than (as it so often is) as though it were written in stone that 'normal value = healthy patient' and the corollary, 'abnormal value = unhealthy patient'.

Who decides what 'normal values' are? Were the samples which provided the raw material for the 'normal values' taken from healthy young patients? If so then there must be a chance that 'normal values' are different for older patients.

There are an infinite number of reasons why a patient could have a result outside 'normal values' and yet be perfectly normal and healthy.

***

The problems associated with tests and investigations are made worse by the fact that doctors undoubtedly order far too many tests. Inevitably, this leads to more false positives – and even more unnecessary treatment.

At least two thirds of all the tests and investigations ordered by hospital doctors and general practitioners are unnecessary.

Routine blood and urine tests help doctors make a diagnosis in only around 1% of cases.

And routine sampling for microbiological testing is often unnecessary. One survey showed that only in 3% of cases was the treatment given based on the result of culture and antibiotic sensitivity.

***

There are several reasons why doctors order too many tests.

1. Tests are sometimes ordered because they provide doctors with some protection from the risk of litigation. A doctor who has bits of paper containing test results to substantiate and support his selected treatment programme will probably be safe from legal action. That is sad but it is a fact of modern life. In countries which have lots of lawyers (you know who you are) the fear of unjustified litigation (fed more by greed than anything else) is very real. But in the long run it is the patients who suffer. Only the lawyers benefit. (As usual.)

2. Unnecessary tests are often ordered to buy doctors time when they don't know what is going on. Doctors who are bewildered or uncertain may simply hide behind technology and order more and more tests in the hope that this scatter gun approach may prove effective. The condition of the patient becomes almost irrelevant as the doctor searches endlessly for the ever elusive diagnosis.

3. Some doctors practise 'hot' or aggressive medicine and insist on collecting all the possible evidence they can even when the diagnosis is not in doubt. This type of doctor will insist on performing an endoscopy so that he can actually see a stomach ulcer even though the patient's history (and, maybe, an X-ray) have made the diagnosis certain.

4. Doctors sometimes order tests to impress their patients, their colleagues, their students or themselves. The more esoteric the test the greater the status associated with its use.

5. It is fairly common these days for doctors to order unnecessary tests because they are planning to write a paper for a scientific journal and need lots of data to fill up the pages and build up their reputations. Most of the papers published in scientific journals are of little or no clinical value and so yet again patients are investigated unnecessarily.

    It is important to remember that just about every procedure (however 'minor' it might appear to be) carries a physical risk. Even sticking a needle into a patient is potentially hazardous and the more complex the procedure the more likely it is that something will go wrong.

    One study showed that 14% of all patients who undergo invasive procedures (such as biopsies, catheterizations or bronchoscopies) have at least one complication. Most complications then need treatment and involve a longer stay in hospital. The longer the patient stays in hospital the more tests are done. And on it goes.

6. Doctors undergo most of their training in hospital. And in teaching hospitals students and young doctors are taught to over-investigate. Consultants frequently berate students who haven't ordered all the possible tests. No attempt is made to decide which tests are likely to prove particularly helpful. No thought is given to the cost of ordering so many tests. And no thought is given to the patient who will spend hours wandering from laboratory to X-ray department and who will end up, in consequence, exsanguinated, irradiated and exhausted.

    The pointlessness of all this was well illustrated by one survey which showed that when bacteriological swabs are taken from patients in hospital there is a two to one chance that the patient will have been discharged before the results of the culture become available. It is, of course, possible that the odd patient may get better before the test results become available but the only sensible conclusion I can draw from this survey is that in most cases the doctor in charge of the patient regards the test that he has ordered as irrelevant to the patient's health.

7. Finally, doctors frequently perform tests out of habit. So for example, patients who are in hospital will often have daily tests done even though a daily change in a specific test is unlikely to lead to a daily change in the treatment recommended. When this happens diagnosis and investigation have been divorced from treatment. The real risk lies in the fact that the more often tests are performed the more likely it is that there will be one or more results showing a new and abnormal result – and that the new, abnormal result will inspire doctors to introduce another element to the treatment programme.

***

Ever since Röntgen first discovered X-rays at the end of the nineteenth century radiology has played an increasingly important part in the average doctor's investigative armamentarium.

Since 1968 medical journals around the world have frequently carried papers pointing out that most X-rays are unnecessary, extremely expensive, potentially hazardous and unlikely to contribute anything to a doctor's knowledge of a patient's illness, to the way that the patient is treated or to his or her long term health. Doctors frequently order X-rays as a comforting ritual rather than for any specific purpose. And, of course, many X-rays are ordered purely for legal protection.

I had good personal experience of the possible danger of an X-ray a few years ago. When an investigative X-ray showed that I had a strangely shaped kidney the two radiologists who had studied the X-ray plates wanted me to see a surgeon. Because of the X-ray they thought I had renal cancer and urgently needed major surgery. After I insisted on another opinion a third radiologist immediately spotted that my abnormal kidney wasn't pathologically abnormal at all. I just happened to have a mis-shaped kidney.

***

Many doctors have become totally dependent on tests of one sort or another. They feel incapable of making any sort of clinical decision unless they have done a vast range of tests. And they put more faith in the results they obtain from the laboratory or the X-ray department than they do in their own clinical skills.

Whenever a doctor plans to do tests or investigations of any sort ask him how they will affect the way he treats you.

If he tells you that the test isn't going to affect the treatment (or lack of it) then the test may not be worth having. It is always worth remembering that tests can cause serious health problems – and can kill.

***

The bottom line is that you should remember that tests aren't as reliable, as useful or as necessary as most people think they are.

If you feel ill when tests have shown that there is nothing wrong with you then you should listen to your body and ignore what may well turn out to be 'false negative' tests.

If you feel well when tests have shown that you have a problem which needs treating just remember that there is a chance that you are feeling well because there isn't anything wrong with you – and that it is the laboratory test equipment rather than your body which needs treatment.

Chapter Twenty

Nine Ways To Save Yourself From Stress

1. Be prepared to admit when you're feeling tired. If you keep going when you're exhausted you'll not only make yourself worse (by doing further damage to your immune system) but you'll also let yourself – and the people around you – down. You can't do your best work when you're suffering from burn out.

2. Learn to manage your time as efficiently as possible. Plan your day. Keep a diary so that important engagements and commitments don't suddenly creep up on you.

3. Beware of stimulants such as caffeine, tobacco or alcohol. You may think that one or more of these substances will help you get through the day but all of them can seriously damage your health and, in the long run, make you more, not less, susceptible to stress and pressure. When you take a drug (and caffeine, tobacco and alcohol are all drugs) you may succeed in covering up the symptoms of stress – but you won't have done anything about the problems causing the stress and you certainly won't have eradicated the symptoms produced by the stress. By continuing to push yourself hard you will be doing an enormous amount of damage to your immune system.

4. If you feel ill take time off. Don't think that you're indispensable and must carry on. The cemeteries are full of people who thought they were indispensable, but life goes on without them. If you feel exhausted then your body is telling you that it needs to rest. Remember that regular holidays are important – and make sure that the holiday you choose is relaxing. Your immune system will automatically repair and rebuild itself when you take a break.

5. If your life is full of battles and arguments make sure that you take time out to relax and enjoy yourself. And make sure too that you differentiate between those battles which are worth fighting and those which are merely adding to the stress in your life. If you learn to walk away from trivial and insignificant problems you will retain your strength for the battles which really matter. Stand up for yourself over important issues but be prepared to walk away from arguments when the underlying issue isn't truly important. People who are always complaining burn themselves out with anger so think very carefully before allowing yourself to get heated up. If the battle is important then do what you think is right – and fight to the last breath if necessary. If the battle isn't important then try to shrug your shoulders and walk away.

6. Physical exercise is a great way to get rid of frustrations, angers and disappointments. But if you haven't done any physical exercise for a long time get yourself back into the swing gently. Make sure that you get professional medical advice before you start an exercise programme and, if you are planning to do anything other than go walking, cycling or swimming take advice from an exercise professional too. And do remember that too much physical exercise can damage your immune system. Top class international athletes frequently suffer from colds and other minor infections because although they may be fit (in the athletic sense) they are not healthy and their immune systems are in poor shape.

7. Make sure that you get enough sleep. If you have difficulty in relaxing at night try having a hot bath before you go to bed. Don't do any work for at least an hour before you try to get to sleep. Watch a relaxing video or read an amusing or entertaining book. Poor sleep is a symptom of burn out – and it makes things steadily worse. Your immune system gets recharged while you're sleeping – as long as you are relaxed.

8. Learn to say 'no' more often. Don't let yourself be tricked into taking on too many responsibilities by people who know how to make you feel guilty. Get your priorities sorted out and remember that you – and your family and friends – need some of your life.

9. Try not to get too upset when things go wrong. Remember that you can't get anywhere in life without taking risks or without making mistakes. Try not to brood over your failures but try to learn from your mistakes. Otherwise your bad days will smoulder and add to your burn out.

Chapter Twenty One

If You Are Contemplating Surgery

If you have to have surgery make sure that the surgeon still performs at least thirty operations a year of the type you need.

And before you agree to have surgery make sure that you know the answers to these questions:

1. What are the alternatives? (Including treatments which do not involve surgery.)
2. What is likely to happen to me if I do not have the operation?
3. What is the overall success rate for this operation?
4. Are there any other operations which might be safer and/or more effective?
5. If you are a pre-menopausal woman ask if the operation is more likely to be a success if you have it done at a particular time in your menstrual cycle.
6. What are possible/likely side effects of the operation?
7. How is the operation going to improve my life?
8. Is the operation really suitable for me?
9. How experienced is the surgeon who is planning to perform the operation? (Ask who is going to perform the operation – the consultant or one of his assistants.)
10. What after care will I need? How long will I need nursing? When can I go home? How long will I need to stay off work?

Chapter Twenty Two

Get Your Timing Right

It has been known for centuries that the leaves of some plants regularly open during the daytime and close at night. It was always assumed that this phenomenon was a response to sunlight. But in 1729, a French astronomer called Jean-Jacques de Mairan, conducted a very simple experiment which showed that this assumption was wrong. He discovered that this phenomenon occurs even if a plant is kept in the dark. The only possible explanation was that the plant opens and closes not according to the changes in the amount of available light but in response to some sort of 24 hour internal clock. That was the first experiment in chronobiology.

Since then chronobiology (the study of temporal patterns related to biological phenomena) has become an acknowledged science. It is now known that just about every living organism – from a nucleated single cell to a human being – follows a 24 hour or circadian rhythm.

Here are just some of the vital observations which have been made about human beings:

♦ Your pulse rate and blood pressure are highest first thing in the morning (with the result that the incidence of heart attack and stroke is highest at that time of day). In the evening your pulse rate and blood pressure will naturally fall.

♦ Your body temperature rises during the day and falls at night.

♦ Blood platelets – which help with blood clotting – are stickier in the morning than at any other time of day. You are, therefore, likely to have less trouble with bleeding if you nick yourself in the morning than if you nick yourself in the evening. (Shaving in the morning is less likely to produce a troublesome cut that won't stop bleeding than shaving in the evening).

♦ Your tolerance for alcohol peaks at five o'clock in the afternoon.

♦ Most babies are born – and most people die – between the hours of midnight and dawn.

♦ The number of white cells in your blood stream (and, therefore, the efficiency of your immune system) fluctuates all the time – with variations of as much as 50% during a single day.

Our bodies respond in a cyclical way because we have evolved on earth – and the amount of light and heat, and the level of electromagnetic and gravitational forces on our planet all vary in a rhythmic way.

The important thing – still widely ignored by doctors and many alternative health care professionals – is that the abnormalities associated with disease also vary in a cyclical and circadian way.

Whether you are suffering from cancer, heart disease, arthritis or asthma your disease will change during the day and, consequently, whatever you do to tackle the disease should also be arranged according to a circadian rhythm. For example, during the day and the night your body's ability to absorb drugs will vary. When given at the right time of day a drug will have a powerful and positive effect on an illness. But when given at the wrong time of day a drug may prove toxic.

Consider allergy reactions.

Allergy reactions develop when the body's natural defences against foreign organisms over-react. If you are exposed to a pollen or a type of food to which you are allergic your body will send white blood cells to the site at which the foreign organisms have been spotted. The white cells will then proceed to eat up the foreign organisms. Some of the white cells release a substance called histamine which increases local blood flow and triggers the release of more white cells. The symptoms produced by this reaction include pain, itchiness, burning, redness and swelling.

Your body's ability to deal with outside threats in this way is influenced by the amount of glucocorticoid (a steroid hormone) in your blood stream. When the amount of glucocorticoid is at its highest your body's ability to deal with an outside organism will be at its lowest.

Now, under the influence of your body's circadian rhythm the amount of glucocorticoid in your blood is at its highest level in the morning – at around 5 or 6 am. Inevitably, therefore, your body's ability to deal with an external threat is lowest at this time of day.

But in the evening when your body's levels of glucocorticoid fall your body's ability to deal with a threat rises.

This means that you are least likely to develop an allergy reaction early in the morning. But, at that same time of day, you are also, because of the same effect, most susceptible to infection.

On the other hand you are most likely to develop an allergy reaction – and least susceptible to infection – in the evening.

Next, consider arthritis – a common inflammatory disease which also runs on a biological clock.

In rheumatoid arthritis the joints are attacked by a malfunctioning immune system. The joints of a rheumatoid arthritis sufferer are usually stiffest and most swollen early in the morning. They become easier during the day. In other types of arthritis – such as osteoarthritis – the stiffness and pain get worse during the day.

It is clear from this knowledge that the time when medication is given for these two different types of disease is vital. A drug given for rheumatoid arthritis should be timed to act in the morning, whereas a drug given for osteoarthritis should be timed to be working most efficiently later in the day.

Asthma is one of the commonest diseases in the world. It is said to be getting commoner.

Because of the circadian rhythms associated with a number of normal physiological processes (such as airway size and breathing patterns) the majority of asthma attacks take place between two and six o'clock in the morning. The airways are open widest during the day and there is a reduction in airflow after midnight (and particularly between two and six in the morning).

Heart disease is linked to body rhythms too. Heart attacks are twice as common in the morning as they are during the rest of the day – making high-stress breakfast meetings a risky venture.

The activity of cancer cells is also linked to body rhythms.

Drugs prescribed to attack cancer usually operate by killing cells when they are most vulnerable – during the process of division. Anti-cancer drugs target cancer cells because cancer cells grow and divide far faster than other human body cells. However, other rapidly dividing cells (particularly cells inside the intestine and cells in the bone marrow) are likely to be killed unnecessarily by anti-cancer drugs.

However, if an anti-cancer drug is given at the right time of day the problems associated with such a drug can be minimised and the effectiveness of the drug can be maximised. One trial showed that women with ovarian cancer who were given their drugs at the right time of day were four times as likely to survive for five years than other women – whose drug taking was not regulated in this way.

Other researchers have found a similar difference when treating patients with colon cancer.

It isn't just drug therapy which is influenced by time. There is evidence which suggests that far more pre-menopausal women survive breast surgery if they have an operation which is done during the second half of their menstrual cycle than if they have an operation in the first two weeks of their cycle. This difference can probably be explained by the change in hormone levels which occurs during a menstrual period.

If researchers put more effort into studies of this sort and wasted less time and money on pointless research such as animal experimentation far more lives would be saved.

The link between surgery, breast cancer, survival rates and the menstrual cycle was first observed in 1836 so I really don't understand why more research hasn't been done to find out the precise link between hormone levels and cancer.

I honestly don't think anyone knows for certain whether or not the time of your operation will really affect your survival chances. But if I was a woman having breast surgery for cancer I would want to have the operation done in the second half of my menstrual cycle.

Any patient who needs drug therapy should ask their doctor to check if there is any evidence to show whether the treatment works best at a particular time of day. My guess is that most doctors will have never heard of chronobiology. But getting the timing right could make a life or death difference so it is well worthwhile being persistent.

This really is an area where more research is needed – and needed fast. It seems to me to be quite absurd that we have failed to pay much attention at all to this absolutely vital branch of medical science. Many deaths and a good deal of illness could be avoided by the expenditure of a relatively small amount of effort in this area.

Timing is vital – for patients as well as for comedians.

Chapter Twenty Three

Listen To Your Instincts When Making Decisions

Do you have difficulty in making decisions? Do you spend hours trying to decide what to wear? Do you spend ages agonising over which item to choose when dining out at a restaurant?

If you're trying to buy a new car/TV set/fridge do you find yourself oscillating helplessly between showrooms, weighed down by facts and quite incapable of coming to any firm conclusion?

There is evidence now to show that looking at all the facts and trying to assess the pros and cons of taking each particular course of action may not be the best way to make a decision.

New research suggests that individuals who suffer from something psychologists call the Hamlet syndrome (introspection combined with indecision) may be able to take a short cut when trying to take decisive action.

Neuroscientists have found that the most successful decision makers are not the ones who agonise over all the evidence, and then assess each new strand of information, before making a decision but those who are in tune with their feelings, who have a good supply of common sense and who have trained themselves to allow their instincts to take over when making decisions.

Making decisions by 'hunch' is, it seems, in the long run more reliable than attempting to analyse all the evidence and all the possible courses of action before coming to a conclusion.

The researchers found that individuals who habitually make a cool, hard assessment of all the facts before making their decisions tend to make self-destructive choices.

(To this, of course, must be added the fact that constantly attempting to make logical, fact based decisions can be extremely time consuming and stressful.)

Although the conclusion that assessing the facts may not be the best way to make decisions undoubtedly sounds surprising, it does fit with the anecdotal evidence I have acquired over the years.

And, after all, listening to all the carefully considered opinions expressed by the so-called experts can get you nowhere. Experts, who invariably claim to base their views on their highly educated and honed skills at interpreting facts frequently disagree and if you ask two experts the same question you can invariably rely on obtaining at least two opposing viewpoints.

There are several possible reasons for this.

First, of course, some of the facts which are used may be of doubtful quality – and may not be 'facts' at all. It is not uncommon for prejudices and assumptions to masquerade as facts. Second, some facts, which may be essential, may be missing. Naturally, you probably won't know that facts are missing if they are not there. And third, it is extremely rare for any expert – however analytical and logical – to be able to interpret facts in an entirely objective manner. Personal prejudices and experiences often get in the way.

Making judgements according to instinct means that, by getting underneath your conscious mind, you are likely to be able to use all the information you have available. Your conscious mind may select and discriminate but your subconscious will have access to every piece of information you have accumulated on the subject.

Instinctive judgements can also be made with relatively little reference to those fears which are such a potent force whenever we are trying to make decisions.

If, when standing in front of your wardrobe, you decide that you will pick out the blue jacket your conscious mind will immediately start to think of all the problems associated with the selection. Some of these problems will be based on past experiences and some will be based on illogical fears. And the more you think about the judgement you have made the greater the number of fears and problems that will spring to mind.

When you decide to abandon your first choice and make a second selection your mind will immediately offer all the reasons why this choice is not a wise one.

In the end you will be quite incapable of making a decision. You will have become a bundle of nerves and you will have wasted a good chunk of your life on a simple and relatively unimportant decision.

When you allow your instincts to take over – and do the decision making for you – you will free yourself from all these problems and enable yourself to make small and big decisions more readily, more accurately and with far less stress and heartache.

167

Now, here is some practical advice on how you can best get in touch with your instincts.

1. If you routinely spend a long time making relatively minor decisions speed up your decision making processes by giving yourself a ten second limit for making decisions. Simply make up your mind to follow whatever thought sprang first into your mind. The chances are high that your first and instinctive decision was the right one. Getting into the habit of relying on your instincts when making minor decisions will have the added benefit of giving you increased confidence in your instinctive decision making ability. (By definition minor decisions don't matter all that much and so the downside – if you make a decision which can later be shown to have been wrong – will be slight. You don't have much to lose but by building up your ability to rely on your instincts you have a great deal to gain.)

2. If you have a difficult problem to solve but find yourself unable to make a decision, give up and do something else. Try to find something completely different – preferably something that will occupy and distract your mind. The chances are high that when you allow your mind to drift back to the original problem an hour or so later you will find that your subconscious mind has continued to work on the problem and has produced a solution.

3. When making instinctive decisions try to relax your body and your mind. Breathe slowly and deeply and close your eyes to cut out all stimulation from the outside world. (Naturally you should forget about the eye closing if you are sitting in your car trying to decide which route to follow – or if you are doing anything which might be hazardous if performed with closed eyes!).

4. When trying to make an instinctive decision ask yourself a specific (rather than a general) question. Don't ask yourself something vague such as: 'How can I be happy?'. And don't confuse your instincts by offering a huge variety of choices all at once. Don't ask yourself: 'Shall I go to France, Italy, Switzerland, Germany or Spain for my holidays this year?' Instead, ask yourself specific questions such as 'Should I take the job as ambassador to France?' 'Should I go to Italy in August?' 'Should I sleep with Dick/Dora?'

5. If you are looking for a solution to a complex, major problem try writing down a list of as many possible answers as you can think of. Scribble down ideas just as quickly as they come into your head. Let your mind roam wherever it wants. Do this for ten or fifteen minutes and then take a close look at what you have written down. You will undoubtedly find that much of what you have written down will look silly or even stupid. The craziest notions can obviously be discarded without

much further attention. But many of the other solutions you have written down will be helpful. One of your jottings may well turn out to be the very solution you have been looking for. At the very least this exercise will give you the chance to examine some previously unexpected options.

6. Do a little practise in order to sharpen up your powers of prediction. Try guessing what will happen tomorrow, next week or next year. Try to decide what the headlines are likely to be over the next few days. Try to decide what is going to happen in politics, in the economy or in forthcoming sporting events. Try to 'see' who wins forthcoming races or competitions. Try to 'see' yourself holding a copy of tomorrow's newspapers – and then try to read the headlines. If you try this technique frequently your brain will become increasingly efficient at sorting out information and producing instant answers. Your intuitive sense will be improved.

Chapter Twenty Four

Learn How To Deal With People Who Make You Feel Inadequate

Is there someone in your life who makes you feel inadequate?

Your mother? Your boss? A sarcastic or manipulative friend?

Do you know someone who always puts you down and makes you feel like a loser? Such people can cause immense physical and mental distress, make you ill and damage your life expectancy.

Here are some quick tips that should help you:

1. Ask them to tell you exactly what they want you to do. People who moan and criticise are often not very good at offering practical advice. Chances are that you will put them on the defensive – you will certainly take the sting out of their attack.
2. Don't let anyone label you unfairly. If someone tells you that you are always unreliable or disorganised give some examples which show that you are just the opposite.
3. Agree with them. This will really take the wind out of their sails.
4. Invade their space. Stand close to them. Most bullies (and this is particularly true of emotional bullies) are cowards. Move closer to them and they'll probably back away – and back down.
5. Ignore them. Say 'thank you' for the advice or comment. And just ignore it.
6. Walk away from potential scenes. Just refuse to get involved in a distressing argument.
7. Avoid people who constantly annoy or upset you. Why waste your life on people who make your life miserable? I don't care who it is – colleague, friend or close relative – if they make you unhappy cut them out of your life.

Chapter Twenty Five

Spend At Least Some Time Living In The Country

People who live in the country live a lot longer than people who live in cities. The differences are big – city dwellers are 66% more likely to die prematurely than country folk – and they are getting bigger.

You might suspect that these differences in life expectation are largely a result of variations in wealth. The poor are, after all, more likely to live in overcrowded conditions in big cities, and more likely to eat an inadequate, fat-rich diet. But wealth is not the primary factor. Even poor people who live in the country frequently live longer than town and city dwellers.

The truth is that many of the lifestyle choices which lead to a longer life are available to everyone – and not dependent on wealth.

Here are the real reasons why living in a city is bad for your health (together with ways in which city dwellers can improve their life expectancy):

1. Despite attempts to reduce pollution the air that is breathed in heavily populated areas is still polluted – largely by cars. There is no easy solution to this problem – masks are uncomfortable and impractical – but regular trips out of town to breathe fresh country air do help. Keeping out of rooms filled with tobacco smoke is also wise. If you have a choice between a ground floor flat and a flat higher up choose the flat higher up – where you are less likely to breathe in concentrated traffic fumes. Remember that breathing through the nose means that the body's natural air filter has a chance to work.

2. People who live in the country are more likely to be able to grow their own (organic) food whereas people who live in cities are more likely to

eat junk food. One reader complained that it is impossible to buy organic food in large cities. This simply isn't true – though organic food may not be available from every supermarket and corner shop it will be available. I don't know of any large city which doesn't have a variety of health food shops where organic food can be purchased. Organic food does cost a little more than junk food. But the difference in cost is more than outweighed by the savings that will be made by not having to purchase vast quantities of patent medicine – and the reduction in earning time lost through ill health.

3. Water pollution contributes to poor health and accelerated mortality rates. People who live in the country are more likely to have their own drinking water supplies (springs, bore holes etc.). People who live in towns and cities should not drink plain tap water (which may contain a variety of chemicals) but should drink only bottled spring water. The cost of drinking clean(er) water is slight. (Filtering tap water helps exclude some chemicals – and makes it safer – but does not exclude all chemicals.)

4. Generally speaking, there is far more stress in cities than there is in the country. Heavy traffic, work pressures and so on conspire to create anxiety. All this means that it is particularly important for city dwellers to learn how to deal with the stress in their lives – and to learn how to increase their resistance to stress. Planning ahead, allowing plenty of time for journeys and deliberately allowing time for relaxation are all ways to minimise the effects of city stress.

5. Loneliness is known to be a major cause of stress, unhappiness and depression in big cities. In small communities people tend to make friends and acquaintances easier than in cities. People moving to cities should join clubs, colleges, associations and so on as soon as possible in order to minimise the effects of loneliness.

6. Noise is a serious cause of stress related health problems among people living in cities. Sound proofing one room may help – as may ear plugs. City centre dwellers who choose third floor (or higher) apartments are less likely to be disturbed by street noise than lower floor inhabitants.

7. Many people who live and work in cities eat while moving or while still working at their desks. Such habits – which are uncommon among country dwellers – are part of the explanation why long term digestive problems are so common among city dwellers.

Chapter Twenty Six

Make Sure You Drink Enough (Water)

Your body needs constant supplies of fresh water and a body which is deprived of water (or not supplied with enough) will soon fall ill. Many women who suffer from frequent urinary infections might suffer less if they drank more water. Water helps to keep muscles in good tone and helps to keep skin looking good.

If you don't drink enough water you will be more likely to suffer from constipation and other bowel disorders such as irritable bowel syndrome. The human body is made up of 75% water and non infectious recurring or chronic pains may suggest that your body needs more fluid.

Drinking water helps to keep your stomach full – and keeps away hunger pangs. So if you don't drink enough water the chances are high that you will feel hungry eat more food than your body needs – and put on excess weight.

Also there is some evidence to show that people who drink plenty of water metabolise stored fat more efficiently. Drinking good amounts of water also helps the body flush out toxins and other waste materials which, if allowed to accumulate, may do harm. Chronic dehydration may well be a fundamental cause of many common diseases.

How much water should you drink? A healthy adult with well functioning kidneys should probably drink six to eight 8 oz. glasses of water a day – I suspect that is far more than most people drink. It is obviously important to make sure that the water is clean, fresh and free from chemical and bacterial contamination.

The water which comes out of your tap – and which may contain chemicals – may not satisfy this requirement unless you filter it first. I wouldn't trust any water company to put chemicals into my drinking water. I believe that the possible risks associated with the addition of fluoride far exceed the benefits. If the people putting the fluoride into the water get the amounts wrong the results can be devastating. Too much fluoride can cause mottling of the teeth, bone disorders and even cancer. Just one person making one mistake could be catastrophic. Are you completely happy that no one working for your water company is ever going to make a mistake? The possibility of fluoride poisoning isn't my only worry about drinking water. Having carefully considered all the evidence I have come to the conclusion that tap water is now unsafe to drink in many areas.

It is also important to remember that drinking lots of tea and coffee or alcohol isn't the same as drinking lots of water. Alcoholic drinks and drinks containing caffeine have a diuretic effect – they induce the body to get rid of water. You can use 'dilute to taste' fruit drinks if you like but I certainly don't recommend that you drink six to eight 8 oz. glasses of fizzy drinks every day. Naturally, if you have a health problem (particularly one which relates to your kidneys) you should talk to your doctor before increasing your fluid intake. You may need to increase your fluid intake slowly, to get your body used to the change. If you drink too much water your kidneys may be unable to cope and your body may retain the fluid.

Chapter Twenty Seven

Before You Travel Ask Yourself If Your Journey Is Really Necessary

If you spend a day sitting in trains or aeroplanes you will probably arrive at your destination feeling exhausted – even though you haven't done anything except sit, eat and read. You may have even noticed that the faster you travel the more exhausted you feel. For example, if you go by plane you may arrive at your destination feeling more worn out than if you travel by train.

There is, I believe, a simple explanation for this.

If you travel with a mobile telephone you will find that the battery wears out far more speedily than normal. The explanation for this phenomenon is that the telephone is constantly searching for new base stations. We know that the human mind is strongly influenced by magnetic fields and that human beings can determine exactly where they are by using magnetic fields. I have a theory (and I admit that it is only a theory) that constant travelling wears out the brain in exactly the same way that constant travelling exhausts the battery of a mobile telephone. When you travel, your brain is constantly working hard to get its bearings. This explains why the faster you travel the more exhausted you get.

If I am right about this then it might, I suppose, be possible to solve the problem by giving trains and aircraft cabins their own magnetic field – with a force slightly stronger than the one normally exerted on the brain. However, interfering with nature in this way could well turn out to be exceedingly dangerous.

My best long term suggestion is a very simple one: travel by train (rather than aeroplane) as often as you can and thereby cut down the speed at which you travel. Travelling by train offers other advantages too: your risk of acquiring an infection will probably be lower (see my book *Superbody*, also published by the European Medical Journal); you can reduce your risk of developing a deep vein thrombosis by walking about occasionally, and the food will probably be better. Travelling by trains also means that you don't have to go through airports – probably the least friendly, most stressful places on earth.

Chapter Twenty Eight

Your Body (And Mind) Need Light And Sunshine To Survive

A friend of mine once complained that for a year his health had been steadily deteriorating. He had difficulty in sleeping, he constantly felt depressed and his wife had complained (and he admitted that he knew it was true) that he had become exceedingly irritable.

There were physical symptoms too. He had acquired an itchy skin rash which had proved to be resistant to everything his doctor could think of prescribing. And he had constant, and exceedingly debilitating, headaches.

There was one pretty clear clue.

The symptoms had started immediately after a move to a new office building. They had disappeared completely during a two week summer holiday. And they had returned immediately after his return to work.

When I told him that I would lay odds that his symptoms were in some way related to his work my friend dismissed the very idea with a firm shake of his head.

Stubbornly he insisted that he enjoyed his work, suffered very little from stress and spent 99% of his working time in a brand new, purpose built office where there could not possibly lurk any unseen dangers to his health.

'I don't work in an out-of-date sweat shop!' he told me, rather proudly – and not a little indignantly. 'It's a state of the art office building. The architects consulted with medical and ergonomic experts. We have, for example, got an incredibly efficient heating and air conditioning system.'

I asked him to invite me to his office so that I could see if I could spot any potential health hazards that he and they might have missed.

177

When I entered my friend's 'state of the art open plan office building' I could hardly believe my eyes.

There were no windows. Not one.

The offices were lit entirely by artificial light and, presumably to save installation and running costs, the building was inadequately supplied with overhead light fittings. Each worker in this twentieth century hive had access to a low wattage multi directional lamp (to reduce eyestrain and improve working efficiency) but there was so little general lighting that my eyes, unaccustomed as they were to the gloom, could hardly see across to the other side of the room.

'I bet your sickness rate has tripled since you moved here,' I said to my friend.

He looked at me, clearly puzzled. 'It has, as a matter of fact. But who told you that?'

'No one,' I replied. 'They didn't have to.' I waved a hand around in the semi-darkness. 'If you carry on working here there is a good chance that you will end up being hospitalised,' I told him quite seriously.

My friend laughed, rather nervously. But he refused to find another job or ask to be transferred. Five months later he was admitted to hospital suffering from severe depression.

The depression was, quite wrongly in my view, attributed to stress. I have no doubt that the depression – and his other symptoms – were caused exclusively by the fact that he spent at least half of his waking life in semi-darkness. During the winter months he spent nearly all his waking life in various stages of gloom.

***

It has been known for centuries that sunlight and artificial light have a powerful impact on both physical and mental health. Hippocrates believed in the therapeutic value of sunlight and for generations afterwards the Greeks accepted this link. But Hippocrates was by no means the first physician to acknowledge the relationship between sunlight and good health. Sunshine was accepted as a healing force in the early civilisation of Mesopotamia.

This long-established truth may be denied or ignored by the cerebrally deficient and drug company sponsored hordes who rule the medical establishment but I would seriously argue that the relationship between light and health has been better proven than most of the poison, slash and burn therapies favoured by orthodox practitioners (which frequently do far more harm than good).

The health benefits of natural sunlight have been used for centuries.

(Surprisingly, many of those doctors who would sneer at the idea that sunlight might have a therapeutic effect would probably not see anything odd in the fact that they regularly tell their patients that the human body can obtain all the vitamin D it needs simply through modest regular exposure of the hands, arms and face to sunlight.)

More recently, in the 1980s, it was established that individuals who are deprived of sunlight may develop a condition called Seasonal Affective Disorder (SAD) – and that the condition can be treated with exposure to light.

***

Could light therapy do more and be used to combat more disorders?

I believe it could. Ultraviolet light is known to have anti-bacterial, anti-viral and anti-fungal properties and there are many who claim that it can be used to help disorders as varied as heart disease, menstrual problems, weak bones, and cancer.

Tragically, however, this low profit therapy (and those who have dared to advocate it) have been dismissed and maligned by the ever powerful medical establishment which, encouraged one presumes by the greedy and enormously unethical pharmaceutical industry, is never enthusiastic about what might be seen as a competitive therapy.

(Governments may have – just about – stopped burning books – although this may be temporary – but they still suppress cures and remedies which threaten the economic success of established forces.)

I would not recommend that sunlight or natural light (or even coloured light) should be regarded as a sole form of therapy for all the disorders which it has been claimed can be helped in this way.

But I do firmly believe that sunlight and natural light are, when combined together with such other factors as a healthy diet, essential for good health and vital in the treatment of disease.

The lesson here is clear: those of us who spend a good deal of time indoors should do everything we can to ensure that we are exposed to as much natural light as possible. Choose a well-lit home over a dark one, keep curtains open as much as possible and spend time outside (while taking the obvious precautions against sun-induced cancers).

Chapter Twenty Nine

The Healing Power of Touch

Back in the 13th century an extremely nasty German Emperor called Frederick II conducted a pretty unforgivably hideous experiment to find out what language children would speak if they were brought up without hearing anyone talking.

If this work had been done during the Second World War, Dr Josef Mengele would have done the research and Hitler would have financed it. If the research was done these days it would be carried out by a university department and paid for by a large international drug company looking for an outlet for a new drug designed to improve linguistic ability.

But Frederick II, a pretty ingenious sadist by anyone's standards, probably had to pay for his ungodly research work out of his own pocket.

The research procedure was simple. He took a number of newborn babies from their parents and gave them to nurses. The nurses were told that they must not touch or talk to the children.

The experiment wasn't much of a success because the babies never grew old enough to learn to talk. Consequently, they never learned a language.

A contemporary authority called Salimbene was almost certainly accurate when he concluded that the babies 'could not live without petting'.

In other words the babies died because they were deprived of human touch.

During the first World War a survey of ten institutions revealed that every baby who was less than two years old had died. Not one baby had survived in any of the institutions.

The babies did not die of infection. And they had been given enough to eat. So what killed them?

Could it have been the fact that all the institutions had introduced a policy (which was strictly followed) that in order to minimise the spread of infectious diseases the babies should be touched as infrequently as possible?

I think it's very likely. In recent years it has become increasingly clear that touching, and being touched, are essential ingredients for a healthy life. (As long as the touching is done in an appropriate way, of course.)

A recent survey showed that premature babies who were given three loving massages every day for ten days gained weight much faster than babies who weren't touched in this way. How much faster? A staggering 47%! The babies who were given the massages left hospital six days sooner than the others – leading to an enormous cash saving for the hospital (or the parents or insurance company).

Hundreds of other studies have shown that infants, children and adults all survive better – and more healthily – if they are given lots of cuddles and touched a great deal. Without physical signs of affection we become more brittle, less emotionally stable and considerably more susceptible to fear, stress and pressure.

It has been shown that babies who are deprived of a close physical relationship become emotionally unstable and develop more slowly than other babies, while children who are deprived of cuddles and hugs become 'harder' and 'tougher' in physical and emotional terms. Eventually they, in turn, will show less affection to those around them.

Moreover, other studies have shown that touching programmes such as massage can help patients suffering from an enormous range of disorders – including depression, diabetes, eating disorders, stress and arthritis.

Now, I can understand why massage may help someone suffering from a muscle disorder. But how can a plain old-fashioned massage possibly help someone suffering from depression?

There obviously can't be any purely physical response.

The only possible conclusion has to be that the massage produces a positive psychological effect which creates a general, body-wide improvement in health. The physical touching (the massage) produces a mental or psychological response which triggers a measurable physical effect.

And that, indeed, has been shown to be the case.

A study of one group of patients found that if they were massaged for just one month there was a significant increase in the number and effectiveness of the natural killer cells in their bodies.

There can be no doubt that touching is a form of healing that works. There are no side effects. It doesn't cost anything. It requires no skill and no training.

But no one can make much profit out of this technique. And so we ignore it.

In my book *Mindpower* (first published 1986 and now published by the European Medical Journal) I advised readers not to be shy about touching other people or allowing people to touch them.

'The word massage has acquired a rather seedy reputation in recent years,' I wrote, 'thanks largely to the fact that it is frequently linked with such words as "topless" and "relief". But a thorough massage can be extremely relaxing and soothing. It can help give us an excuse to touch one another. And it certainly can be therapeutic.'

I pointed out in that same book that it is sometimes possible to soothe a troubled individual to sleep by gently massaging his or her forearm with a single finger.

As a junior hospital doctor I often used this simple technique with remarkable success when I was helping to look after elderly patients or small babies who couldn't rest or get to sleep. My theory was, and is, that this simple technique worked best with people at either end of the age spectrum because they were least likely to be offended, embarrassed or shocked.

Researchers all around the world have shown that we can all benefit from a warm, caring relationship – and that simple physical expressions of our caring can be therapeutic. Insurance companies have shown that if a wife kisses her husband goodbye when he sets off to work in the morning he will be less likely to have a car accident on the way to his office or factory. Amazingly, men who get a morning kiss (and a half-hearted peck on the cheek isn't as good as a proper kiss) live five years longer than men who don't get that morning kiss.

Despite all this evidence (much of which has been available for a number of years now) doctors have done little or nothing to encourage patients to take advantage of this facility for healing.

(Cynics will argue – and, as I have already suggested, I would find it difficult to disagree with them – that touching isn't promoted or even discussed because no one has worked out how to make much of a profit out of it.)

***

One of my favourite hobbies is sitting in cafés 'people watching'.

An American psychologist who tried this noticed that there are vast differences between the number of times people in different cities touch one another.

In Puerto Rico a couple will touch one another 180 times an hour. In Paris couples touch 110 times an hour. In the US the figure is two. Yes, couples in America touched one another just twice in an hour. And in London? Zero. Nought. Never. The reserved British hardly ever touch one another in public. (And they don't touch one another very much in private either.) It is hardly surprising that stress-related diseases seem to be commoner in Britain than anywhere else in the world.

In many mainland European countries people are constantly touching one another – even if it is only to shake hands or pat one another on the arm or shoulder. In France friends kiss one another on the cheek when they meet and when they part. Become a 'regular' in a French café and the waiter and the patron will rush to shake you by the hand when you walk in. The Americans and the British, overcome by reserve and political correctness, shy away from touching one another at all.

***

We should all take advantage of the power of touch. Touch other people as often as you can. And encourage them to touch you too. Get someone else to give you a manicure or a shampoo or a massage. Kiss and hug your close relatives when you see them and when you say goodbye to them. And remember that it is just as important that you do not shy away when someone who is close to you approaches with a kiss, a hug or some other physical sign of affection. Try to get rid of old-fashioned prejudices against showing affection in public. Some people still think it is wrong for couples to hold hands or exchange kisses in the street. What nonsense! Whatever your age you are never too old (or too young) to hold hands in public.

These prejudices against touching are based on an unhealthy mixture of guilt and unnatural embarrassment.

Touching someone shows them that you care. Done gently and with affection it is the physical manifestation of loving and caring. It could prolong your life by several years. And, together with a low fat vegetarian diet, an effective approach to stress management and regular gentle exercise, it could well help you overcome at least some existing health problems as effectively (and more safely) as anything the modern medical profession has to offer.

Chapter Thirty

Learn How To Navigate Life's Rock Strewn Passageways

Have you noticed that every small company seems to have a mission statement these days? Your local cobbler probably has one tacked up above the counter. Even the local café probably has one.

Having a mission sounds pretty corny. And it is true that many of the commercial ones are trite, pretentious and false, and born out of commercial expediency rather than a passionate yearning to do what is right.

But there is good sense in having your own mission statement: a map for life; a small collection of very personal guidelines designed to help you navigate life's rock strewn passageways.

Simply earning a living isn't reason enough to get up and go to work. And keeping up with the dull, predictable antics of TV soap characters isn't the sort of driving purpose which will give your life real meaning.

Most people spend their lives being battered around by circumstances; rarely, if ever, in control of their own lives or their destinies.

Time and effort is wasted collecting material stuff which has no lasting worth and which provides little more than transient satisfaction.

To have a sense of worth, a sense of identity and a feeling of genuine self esteem you must identify the things which are really important to you.

Here are some pretty basic questions that you may not have asked yourself very often in the past:

- What would you die for?
- What do you live for?
- What do you want to achieve with your life?
- Do you want to be remembered for what you are doing with your life now?

- If you die tomorrow will you have made full use of your talents?
- Will you have realised your potential?
- How long is it since you asked yourself really searching questions about what you really stand for?
- How much of your life do you fritter away on trivial and inconsequential activities – while the really important things (the things which will make a difference to you and to other people) are put to one side and eventually forgotten?

You can give your life solid principles for the future – and a mission to ensure that you always know exactly where you are heading and why.

Here are my eleven suggestions – a team of principles and proposals designed to help give your life meaning and purpose and to provide you with a stable base in a very wobbly world. These are very personal suggestions. You may feel that some of them are inappropriate. You may not like any of them. But, hopefully, you will feel that they trigger off some thoughts of your own.

1. Get to know yourself. Understand what you really want out of life. And learn to respect yourself and others. If you respect yourself then you have a right to expect others to respect you too. How can you possibly expect other people to respect you if you don't even respect yourself? Remember that courtesy is an important way of showing respect.

2. Spend your time carefully – remembering that time is the most valuable commodity any of us have. The things which matter most to you should not be at the mercy of things which matter not at all. It is easy to put off the important things and to fritter away the hours on trivia. Into every life must come some trivia. And these days the trivia rains down in bucketfuls. Whoever you are, wherever you work, however you would like to spend your days, you will find yourself dealing with bureaucracy, with forms and with pointless paperwork. Some of the trivia is unavoidable. But much of it you can ignore. Or you can, at least, determine to give the important things in your life precedence over the trivia. Never forget that when you sell (or give away) your time you are selling (or giving away) part of your life.

3. Give yourself short, medium and long term targets. Decide where you want to go to in your life and where you want to be in five, ten and twenty years time. Without a map there is a risk that you will wander around aimlessly; frittering away your days, your months and eventually your life. Remember that you cannot possibly begin to live properly until you have found something for which you would die.

4. Say 'no' to the unimportant things. Every day you have to say 'no' to

something. Make sure you say 'no' to the things which don't matter. Remember that every choice involves a cost.

5. Stand up for those who are weaker or more vulnerable than you are. Bullying and cruelty are abhorrent and when we say nothing we dishonour ourselves. Remember that cruelty to animals is just as unforgivable as cruelty to human beings.

6. Be aware that the way you see the problem is the problem. What matters is not so much what we experience but how we respond to our experiences.

7. Never stop learning. Strive constantly to improve the skills you have and to acquire new skills. And remember that if you learn from your mistakes then they help you grow stronger. Remember to remain sceptical when confronted with claims made for new products, treatments or cures. It is becoming increasingly difficult to separate the honest from the dishonest. The more you know the more you will be able to spot the dishonest.

8. Concentrate your efforts on those areas where you can have influence. And gradually try to expand the extent of your influence. Do not make the mistake of thinking that you are without influence. You can have all the influence you want.

9. Learn to understand other people's needs and fears. When you listen to someone try to understand things from their point of view. Do not try to see their problem through your eyes, and do not rush in with advice before you understand their needs and fears.

10. Allow your conscience to speak to you. And learn to listen. Never compromise with your principles. Your principles are what you are. They define you. Focus on your principles and let them run your life.

11. Remember that the best, simplest and easiest question to ask yourself is: 'Why?' Ask it when you are about to move house, take a new job or take on any new responsibility. 'Why do you want to buy a holiday home?' 'Why do you want to buy a new car?' Only when you ask yourself 'Why?' will you know what you really need and what you are prepared to do for it. Most people earn and spend without ever asking themselves 'Why?'.

Ask yourself 'Why?' more often and you will learn more about yourself and about what you are doing with your life. And your longer, healthier life will be a fuller, happier one too.

For a catalogue of Vernon Coleman's books
please write to:

Publishing House
Trinity Place
Barnstaple
Devon EX32 9HJ
England

Telephone	01271 328892
Fax	01271 328768

Outside the UK:

Telephone	+44 1271 328892
Fax	+44 1271 328768

Or visit our websites:

www.vernoncoleman.com
www.lookingforapresent.com
www.makeyourselfbetter.net

Other books by Vernon Coleman

Bodypower

The secret of self-healing

A new edition of the sensational book which hit the *Sunday Times* bestseller list and *The Bookseller* Top Ten Chart.

This international bestseller shows you how you can harness your body's amazing powers to help you conquer 9 out of 10 illnesses without seeing a doctor.

The book also covers:

- How your personality affects your health
- How to stay slim for life
- How to break bad habits
- How to relax your body and mind
- How to improve your figure
- And much much more

'Don't miss it. Dr Coleman's theories could change your life'
(SUNDAY MIRROR)

'A marvellously succinct and simple account of how the body can heal itself without resorting to drugs'
(THE SPECTATOR)

'Could make stress a thing of the past'
(WOMAN'S WORLD)

Paperback £9.95

Published by European Medical Journal
Order from Publishing House • Trinity Place • Barnstaple • Devon
EX32 9HJ • England
Telephone 01271 328892 • Fax 01271 328768

Other books by Vernon Coleman

Mindpower

How to use your mind to heal your body

A new edition of this best-selling book which explains how you can use your mental powers for improving and maintaining your health. Topics covered include:

- How your mind influences your body
- How to control destructive emotions
- How to deal with guilt
- How to harness positive emotions
- How daydreaming can relax your mind
- How to use your personal strengths
- How to conquer your weaknesses
- How to teach yourself mental self defence
- Specific advice to help you enjoy good health
- And much, much more

What they said about the first edition:

'Dr Coleman explains the importance of mental attitude in controlling and treating illness, and suggests some easy-to-learn techniques.' (WOMAN'S WORLD)

'An insight into the most powerful healing agent in the world – the power of the mind.' (BIRMINGHAM POST)

'Based on an inspiring message of hope.' (WESTERN MORNING NEWS)

'It will be another bestseller.' (NURSING TIMES)

Paperback £12.95

Published by European Medical Journal
Order from Publishing House • Trinity Place • Barnstaple • Devon
EX32 9HJ • England
Telephone 01271 328892 • Fax 01271 328768

Other books by Vernon Coleman

Spiritpower

Discover your spiritual strength

This inspirational book will help you rediscover your life's dreams
and help you fulfil your ambitions. Also includes:

- Find out who you are (and what you want)
- Three words that can change your life
- How to get what you want out of life
- Use your imagination and your subconscious mind
- Why you have more power than you think you have
- How you can control your own health
- Why you shouldn't be afraid to be a rebel
- How to stand up for yourself
- Know your fears and learn how to conquer them

What the papers say about *Spiritpower*:

'The final tome in his trilogy which has produced the bestsellers
Bodypower and *Mindpower*, this is Dr Coleman's assessment of our
current spiritual environment, and his prescriptions for change.
He advises both awareness and rebellion, recommending ways to
regain personal autonomy and fulfilment.'
(THE GOOD BOOK GUIDE)

'*Spiritpower* will show you how to find freedom and give meaning
to your life.' (SCUNTHORPE EVENING TELEGRAPH)

'This is a handbook for tomorrow's revolutionaries. Dr Coleman
offers an understanding of the society we live in, in order to show
where our freedom was lost.' (GREENOCK TELEGRAPH)

paperback £12.95

Published by European Medical Journal
Order from Publishing House • Trinity Place • Barnstaple • Devon
EX32 9HJ • England
Telephone 01271 328892 • Fax 01271 328768

Other books by Vernon Coleman

How To Overcome Toxic Stress and the Twenty-First Century Blues

If you are frustrated, bored, lonely, angry, sad, tired, listless, fright-ened, unhappy or tearful then it is possible that you are suffering from Toxic Stress.

After three decades of research Dr Coleman has come up with his own antidote to Toxic Stress which he shares with you in this inspirational book. In order to feel well and happy again you need to take a close look at your life and put things back in the right order. Dr Coleman shows you how to value the worthwhile things in life and give less time to things which matter very little at all.

The book contains hundreds of practical tips on how to cope with the stresses and strains of daily life.

'Never have I read a book that is so startlingly true. I was dumb-founded by your wisdom. You will go down in history as one of the truly great health reformers of our time.'
(EXTRACTED FROM A LETTER TO THE AUTHOR)

'This book is absolutely outstanding ... it addresses a serious problem which up until now has not been identified or discussed in any meaningful way. If you feel you have a lot of stress being generated from outside your life, this book is an absolute must. Personally, I am going to get five copies so that I can put them in my lending library and lend them to as many people as I can.'
(HEALTH CONSCIOUSNESS, USA)

paperback £9.95

Published by European Medical Journal
Order from Publishing House • Trinity Place • Barnstaple • Devon
EX32 9HJ • England
Telephone 01271 328892 • Fax 01271 328768